Expert praise for

Natural Health for African Americans!

"Drs. Walker and Singleton have created a unique
and comprehensive plan that brings the many benefits
of natural health to this neglected audience."
—Mark Mayell, former editor of
Natural Health magazine

"Enjoyable, easy to read . . . a wonderful, holistic approach. . . .
A great handbook for African American health."
—Gwen Rowe-Lee, executive director,
Bay Area Black Consortium
for Quality Health Care, Inc.

"A must-read for physicians. . . . The longest journey begins
with a single step—this is the place to start."
—Leon E. Brown, M.D., diplomate of the
American Board of Dermatology

"Provides important traditional health care information of
particular relevance to the African American population."
—Jose E. Carneiro, Ed.D.,
international health consultant

Natural Health for African Americans

THE PHYSICIANS' GUIDE

Marcellus A. Walker, M.D.
and
Kenneth B. Singleton, M.D.

A LYNN SONBERG BOOK

WARNER BOOKS

A Time Warner Company

A LYNN SONBERG BOOK

IMPORTANT NOTE: Neither this nor any other book should be used as a substitute for professional medical care or treatment. It is advisable to seek the guidance of a physician or other qualified health practitioner before implementing any of the approaches to health suggested in this book. This book was written to provide selected information to the public concerning conventional and alternative medical treatments. Research in this field is ongoing and subject to interpretation. Although we have made all reasonable efforts to include the most up-to-date and accurate information in this book, there is no guarantee that what we know about the subjects discussed in this book won't change with time. The reader should bear in mind that this book is not intended to take the place of medical advice from a trained medical professional. Readers are advised to consult a physician or other qualified health professional regarding treatment of all their health problems. Neither the publisher, the producer, nor the authors take any responsibility for any possible consequences from any treatment, action, or application of medicine or preparation by any person reading or following the information in this book.

Grateful acknowledgment is given to Alcoholics Anonymous World Services, Inc., for permission to reprint on page 203 an excerpt from the booklet *Is AA for You?*

Warner Books, Inc., 1271 Avenue of the Americas, New York, NY 10020

Visit our Web site at http://warnerbooks.com

A Time Warner Company

Printed in the United States of America
First Printing: February 1999
10 9 8 7 6

Library of Congress Cataloging-in-Publication Data
Walker, Marcellus A.
    Natural health for African Americans : the physicians' guide / Marcellus A. Walker and Kenneth B. Singleton.
        p.   cm.
    ISBN 0-446-67369-2
    1. Afro-Americans—Health and hygiene. 2. Holistic medicine.
3. Consumer education.   I. Singleton, Kenneth B.   II. Title.
RA448.5.N4W35   1998
613'.089'96073—dc21   98-24371
                                                                          CIP

Cover design by Christian Van Bree
Book design and text composition by Nancy Singer Olaguera

The greatest gift we can do for others is not to share our riches with them, but to reveal their riches to themselves.
Anonymous

I dedicate this book to all of the teachers of the world, and to the student that is in all of us. I further dedicate this book to my wife, my parents, and my family. Lastly, I dedicate this book to you; may it bring you joy and the hope of new possibilities.
—*M.A.W.*

I dedicate this book to my parents, Harold and Mary Singleton, who have inspired my spiritual growth to greater heights through their humble and prayerful example. And to my son, Marcus, who has taught me the true meaning of being human. And finally to Janelle Goetcheus, M.D., the best physician I know.
—*K.B.S.*

Acknowledgments

We could not have written this book without the inspiration and input of a number of friends and colleagues. We want to offer our special thanks to Jeffrey Bland, Alex Cadoux, Winifred Conkling, Marilyn Dimas, Carolyn Myss, Alvin and Gloria Singleton, Dwight Singleton, Joy Tyson, Christina Walker, Len Wisneski, and Paul Yanick. In addition, we offer thanks to our teachers at University of Santa Monica, Howard University, and Johns Hopkins School of Public Health.

Contents

▼

Introduction

▼

While we would like to think that all people are created equal, we are not, at least when it comes to our health. Each of us has a unique genetic and cultural heritage that makes us more—or less—susceptible to certain illnesses and medical conditions. While we can thank our parents for our individual genetic inheritance, as African Americans we share not only a common history, but some common health traits as well.

Unfortunately, to be black in America is to be at a medical disadvantage compared to people of other races. As a group, African Americans suffer disproportionately from serious, chronic illnesses, including heart disease, cancer, stroke, liver disease, diabetes, respiratory disease, and AIDS. All too often, mainstream medical doctors don't understand or appreciate the subtle but important differences between their black and nonblack patients. Rather than treat the unique needs of the individual, many physicians use a one-size-fits-all approach to healing that does not address the special health care needs of their African American patients.

We have seen firsthand the limitations and failures of conventional, Western medicine in the treatment of African Americans. We have seen too many members of our community die prematurely of preventable and controllable diseases. As physicians who have been trained as conventional medical doctors as well as practitioners of natural medicine, we know there is a better way of healing. Our decades of experience working with African American patients have taught us that the best approach to overall health is a combination of conventional, mainstream medicine and natural or "alternative" healing techniques.

Our hopeful health message is that by using a comprehensive, integrated, East-meets-West approach to overall health, African Americans can lower their susceptibility to illness and live longer, healthier lives. As you make your way through this book, you will see there are many things you can do to empower yourself to stay healthy and live a longer, disease-free life. The intention of this book is to outline some of the ways you can begin to optimize your overall health.

THE WHOLE IS GREATER

Natural medicine differs from mainstream medicine in its basic approach to healing. Simply put, conventional medicine treats and manages the symptoms of disease (it strives to make you feel better), while natural medicine treats the whole person—mind, emotions, body, and spirit (it strives to make you well by getting at the root cause of the problem). Natural medicine puts an emphasis on preventing disease, while conventional medicine has only recently begun to appreciate the link between lifestyle choices and overall health.

Natural medicine is based on the simple but profound premise that the human body is designed to heal itself. The practitioner's role is to help the body heal itself, sometimes through the use of nontoxic and natural herbs, supplements, or other treatments. We are truly complementary physicians—in our practices we use both conventional and alternative techniques—but we prefer to use noninvasive, natural methods whenever possible.

We believe that to promote overall health, the practitioner must view the body holistically: The health care provider must focus on the condition of the entire patient, not just the part that is injured or sick. The practitioner must consider not just the body, but the complex interactions of mind, spirit, and body. In contrast, conventional physicians tend to focus their efforts on controlling or suppressing the symptoms of disease or in using drugs or surgery to manage illness, rather than discovering and addressing the root cause, even if it is emotional or spiritual. Conventional physicians look for healing outside the body; natural healers help the patient heal from within.

As practitioners of natural medicine, we recognize that the body has an entire energy system that has not been understood or fully explored by conventional medical doctors. This energy system is precisely and beautifully put together, and in our personal experience, can offer powerful results in preventing illness and treating disease. We believe that treating the energy system of the body can often yield more dramatic results than many of the traditional approaches to health and healing. The key is to be able to see the signals that the body provides by reading them with a new set of glasses. With this change in perspective, a world of possibilities can come forward. Natural medicine is a new way of viewing the body that offers renewed hope for health and healing.

Natural medicine depends on a commitment to health by the individual; it requires the patient to take responsibility for his or her health by adopting a healthy attitude, lifestyle, and diet. The truth is that you cannot mistreat your body by eating an inappropriate diet, avoiding exercise, and engaging in unhealthy habits, then expect to pop a pill or look to another quick fix to make things better when they go wrong (and they will).

In many ways, natural healing is a commonsense approach to health. And in recent years, a growing number of Americans have rediscovered its many benefits. Disillusioned with the invasiveness—and often the ineffectiveness—of many conventional treatments, many open-minded people have turned to practitioners of natural medicine for a new point of view.

No doubt about it, allopathic medicine (the term used to describe conventional Western medicine) is superb at dealing with trauma and bacterial infections, but it is not nearly as effective as natural medicine at managing chronic pain, autoimmune disease, and degenerative conditions. Because of the limitations of conventional medicine, natural medicine has come in vogue. In fact, a 1993 study published in the *New England Journal of Medicine* reported that an astounding one out of every three respondents to their survey had consulted with at least one herbalist, homeopath, dietary counselor, or other practitioner of natural medicine in 1990.

HOW A COUPLE OF AFRICAN AMERICAN M.D.s BECAME NATURAL "HEALERS"

As African American physicians, we both underwent mainstream medical training, Dr. Walker at University of Illinois School of Medicine and Duke University, and Dr. Singleton at Howard University College of Medicine and the Johns Hopkins University School of Hygiene and Public Health.

During medical school, we both remained curious about alternative methods of healing that weren't covered in our medical textbooks. We were both profoundly concerned by the failure of traditional medicine to meet the needs of our people. As medical students, we learned that African Americans die younger and suffer more serious illness than people of other racial groups, but little thought was given as to why this was so or how to reverse these trends.

▼▼▼▼▼▼▼▼▼▼▼▼▼▼▼▼▼▼▼▼▼▼▼▼▼

DR. WALKER'S PHILOSOPHY OF HEALING

In my first year in medical school, I was curious about different methods of natural healing. Above my desk I displayed two posters—one on reflexology and another on Chinese herbs—just to remind me of the alternative approaches to healing that went beyond mainstream medicine. At that time, I instinctively knew that there were spiritual parts of ourselves that played a critical role in health and healing. We cannot divorce the body and the spirit.

I believe that the problem with conventional medicine is that it is based on sameness, not uniqueness. Doctors want to treat all patients the same way, using the same techniques, the same drugs, the same prescriptions. But this approach is fundamentally flawed because we are all individuals, and we need customized treatment to get to the source of our medical problems. Like it or not, physical, spiritual, mental, and emotional factors all contribute to disease. To make a permanent change in health, to transform the patient, we must understand the patient as a unique individual with unique needs.

I have always been able to work within the mainstream medical community—and at the same time move beyond it. The part of me that has been an outsider has left me hungry to learn more and ask more questions. Throughout my career, I have continued to study different natural healing techniques, from acupuncture to herbalism to spiritual psychology. My experience has taught me that these approaches not only work, but they provide a multidimensional approach to healing that makes much more sense than the mainstream mend-and-medicate medical philosophy.

The natural healing techniques I have studied have helped me see a broader horizon of health care. They have shown me a new set of rules that control health and healing, and they open up a new avenue of hope, which I look forward to sharing with you.

▲▲▲▲▲▲▲▲▲▲▲▲▲▲▲▲▲▲▲▲▲▲▲▲▲▲▲▲▲

▼▼▼▼▼▼▼▼▼▼▼▼▼▼▼▼▼▼▼▼▼▼▼▼▼▼▼▼

DR. SINGLETON'S PHILOSOPHY OF HEALING

I felt transformed during my medical training by what I learned about the plight of inner-city African Americans. I saw people dying of preventable diseases, people dying at much younger than normal ages. I saw blacks developing cancer of the pancreas in their thirties and suffering fatal strokes in their forties. I met black patients who would not go to the hospital when they were sick because they believed that you go to the hospital to die. Distrust of doctors was widespread in the African American community. Even black doctors were suspect because it was believed that if they were smart and competent enough, they would be out in the suburbs making lots of money with the white doctors.

Add to this depressing social backdrop a series of devastating lifestyle factors. As a medical student, I believed many of the health problems were created by nutritional deficiencies, so I took every course offered on diet and nutrition. In my work in the community, I found that African Americans suffered from widespread obesity, hypertension, and diabetes. They also ate high-fat, low-fiber foods that failed to meet their basic nutritional needs. In the end, I was surprised not so much by the high rate of disease as by the fact that so many African Americans lived as long as they did on such a deficient and destructive diet and considering many of their negative lifestyle choices.

While my initial interest in natural healing revolved around nutrition and nutritional supplements, I have always remained open to alternative treatments. I believe that every health problem is complex and multifactorial; one size doesn't fit all.

Unless you're willing to look at a health problem holistically, you're not going to come up with a solution that will really work. You need to be open to looking at psychological factors (such as stress and anxiety), spiritual factors (such as faith and personal integrity), and physical factors (such as lifestyle, nutrition, and exercise).

▲▲▲▲▲▲▲▲▲▲▲▲▲▲▲▲▲▲▲▲▲▲▲▲▲▲▲▲

Together, we share a vision of health care for African Americans that includes the use of both conventional and alternative treatments. As medical doctors with extensive training in alternative medicine, we each bring a great deal of clinical experience and specialized knowledge in different healing arts.

USING THIS BOOK

It is our intention with this book to help you take control and optimize your health. We present both the knowledge we have learned from years of scientific study as well as the knowledge we have learned from years of treating thousands of patients. We see this book as an opportunity to introduce you to many ideas that you may not have had an opportunity to think about.

This book can teach you about the important relationships between your heritage and your health. It is built around three central themes:

- **We must redefine what it means to be healthy.** True health involves the mind, body, spirit, and soul. We must see our overall health as an integrated system in which we are more than the sum of our physical complaints and medical symptoms. The chapters in Part 1, "A New Approach to Health," cover these topics.
- **We must learn to nurture ourselves.** African Americans—indeed, all Americans—need to learn how to manage stress, eat right, exercise regularly, and take care of their overall health. We

want to help you make lifestyle adjustments so that you can take care of yourself. Self-care is not selfish; only by nurturing ourselves will we be able to nurture others. Part 2, "Nurturing Ourselves," offers practical advice on healthy living.

- **We must learn to heal ourselves.** Whether the issue is substance abuse, cardiovascular disease, diabetes, or any of a number of other common medical conditions, we must take responsibility for our health, seeking appropriate treatments for our unique medical needs as African Americans. Part 3, "Healing Ourselves," includes six chapters with very concrete and specific advice on how to use natural medicine to manage our particular health care needs. Of course, the information presented here should not replace professional medical care or treatment.

The techniques you will learn here can help you move into alignment with yourself. How many times have you gone for medical help and still not felt quite right after treatment? There is an internal voice in each of us that knows when we are in alignment. Part of the natural medicine process is to help you get in touch with your inner knowing and to honor it.

Our initial word of advice is to view your personal healing as a process. You must start where you are and then move into a new space of living as you become more aware of how to use the techniques of natural healing. You must begin at the beginning, and in this book the road will be laid out before you. Take the first step, and the ground will come up to meet you.

PART I

A New Approach to Health

1

▼

Our Health Profile

The Health Crisis in the African American Community

In our age of "political correctness," many people consider it inappropriate to separate people on the basis of race. But, however unpopular it may be, when it comes to health, race really does matter. It matters because African Americans are more likely than people of other races to die a premature death. According to the statisticians, there is an 8.5-year difference in the median survival rate between white and black males and a 5.9-year gap between white and black females.

And our health status is getting worse. While the health profile of other ethnic groups is improving, the prognosis for African Americans is deteriorating. A study reported in the *American Journal of Public Health* found that the gap in the life expectancy between blacks and whites grew in the late 1980s. Since the turn of the century, life expectancy at birth in the United States has generally increased for all races. But from 1984 to 1989 life expectancy for whites increased, while life expectancy for blacks decreased. Never before had this pattern occurred in the United States over a sustained period. Why? For black males, the most significant factors were an increase in HIV infection and homicide. For black females, the spread of HIV infection, diabetes, and pneumonia contributed to the death toll.

In addition to the difference in death rates, African Americans also

3

suffer more often than other races from both chronic and acute illness. Consider the grim statistics:

- Heart disease: The age-adjusted death rates from heart disease were 27 percent greater in black men than white men and a remarkable 55 percent higher in black women than white women.

- Diabetes: An estimated three million African Americans have diabetes, which adds up to one in every ten of us. We are 55 percent more likely than whites to have diabetes; the disease is especially prevalent in older black women.

- Lupus: Of the more than 500,000 people stricken with lupus, nine out of ten are women ages fifteen to forty-five—and three out of five are black.

- Sickle cell trait: This condition strikes one out of twelve of us; it occurs to a lesser degree among southern Italians, Greeks, East Indians, and Hispanic people.

- Infertility: African Americans are affected by infertility nearly 1½ times more often than whites.

- AIDS: African Americans and Latinos together total 21 percent of the population, but they account for 46 percent of the U.S. AIDS cases so far. AIDS is now the tenth leading cause of death nationwide for people of all races.

- Hypertension: High blood pressure is twice as common in blacks as in whites, affecting one in three of us.

- Infant mortality: Our children are twice as likely as white children to die before their first birthday. For each 1000 black babies born in the United States, nineteen die by age one, compared with eight of 1000 white babies. That pattern has existed for more than forty years.

- Cancer: African Americans develop cancer about 10 percent more often than the general population, and our mortality rates are 20 to 40 percent higher. One of the key reasons for our poor mortality rate is that our cancer is often undetected until it reaches a more advanced—and less curable—stage. At each stage of discovery, African Americans don't do as well as their white counterparts. Our overall poor diet also plays a major role in our high cancer rate.

- Addiction: African Americans accounted for 39 percent of the drug abuse–related emergency room visits reported to the Drug Abuse Warning Network of the National Institute on Drug Abuse in 1988. Fully 70 to 75 percent of the nation's 2 to 2½ million heroin addicts are black.

These numbers can be numbing, but, as we have seen time and again through our work with African Americans, such statistics are more than abstractions: They represent real people. Every day patients enter our offices with illnesses and medical conditions that can—and should—be prevented or controlled.

Some studies have actually estimated that at least 75,000 African Americans die each year of manageable diseases. In 1985, the U.S. Department of Health and Human Services released *The Report of the Secretary's Task Force on Black and Minority Health*, an eight-volume work based on the federal government's study of the health status of American minority groups. These reports documented what had been presumed for a long time: The gap in health status between white and black Americans was very significant. This led the secretary to conclude that more than 60,000 excess deaths occurred per year for blacks compared to the general population. (Follow-up research found that the number had jumped to 75,000 deaths by 1993.) While researchers have proved that being African American brings myriad health problems with it, the most significant question for the individual becomes, What can I do about it?

BEATING THE ODDS

Fortunately, you can change the odds—and perhaps even beat the odds—by taking care of yourself. However, we have found that in the past twenty-five years or so, the lifestyles of blacks in this country have actually become more unhealthy. African Americans tend to exercise less and eat more junk foods than we used to; we drink sugared soda rather than pure water; we structure our lives so that we have many stresses and few avenues to relieve that stress.

While the current health statistics look depressing, we believe that if we don't take better care of ourselves, African Americans (as well as people of other races) will soon experience an epidemic of cancer, fibromyalgia, chronic fatigue, and other degenerative diseases. It's inevitable: The years of unhealthy living will someday take their toll on people now in their thirties and forties. Such comments, of course, apply to the population in general. As an individual, you have the ability to make healthy food choices, to exercise regularly, to practice stress-reduction techniques, and to improve your overall lifestyle.

Even relatively minor changes can make a major difference in your overall health. Consider the example of Thelma, a fifty-one-year-old with high blood pressure who came to us for help managing her condition. Her blood pressure averaged 160/100, she was thirty-two pounds overweight, and she had a family history of diabetes. She craved sugars and starches, though her blood sugar levels remained normal. We designed a diet program for her that eliminated sugar and white flour without limiting her calories significantly. She participated in an exercise program and ate a low-sodium diet; she lost an average of two pounds per week and within several months her blood pressure dropped to 130/86—within the normal range—without resorting to the use of antihypertensive drugs. As Thelma reminds us, a healthier lifestyle doesn't have to entail great hardship and deprivation, just the establishment of new, more healthful lifestyle choices.

GET MOTIVATED

Chances are good that you have a long list of lifestyle changes that you know you should make but you haven't put them into effect quite yet. You know you should eat at least five servings of fruits and vegetables a day. You know you should eat a high-fiber, low–animal fat diet, and give up junk foods. You know you should exercise regularly, give up the cigarettes, limit the alcohol. You know you should find healthy ways of letting go of stress and relaxing when tensions arise. You know you should avoid excessive sun exposure, get plenty of rest, and drink plenty of water every day.

But the chances are good you aren't doing all the good things you should to take care of yourself. The problem: motivation.

When it comes to motivation and sticking to a program for health, we have found that our patients tend to fall into one of three categories. One group—about 15 percent of our patients—immediately apply the health information, even if it requires making difficult lifestyle adjustments. A second group of 15 percent or so never will embrace the information and put it into practice, no matter what you tell them. (These are the people who refuse to quit smoking even after they've been diagnosed with lung cancer. Of course, we each have the right to make our own choices about how we will care for our own body.) The third group, the 70 percent in the middle, want to do the right thing but need a little extra motivation. Our challenge as physicians is not just to introduce our patients to natural medicine and to offer prescriptive advice, but also to use our experience as healers to help encourage people to put the knowledge into action.

While there is often a temptation to use fear of disease as a motivator, it rarely works as a powerful enough incentive to support lifelong change. Sometimes fear can help get someone started eating right or exercising or meditating, but fear diminishes over time. It is difficult for a person to internalize the message and firmly establish good habits before finding a way to rationalize changing back to their old ways.

Rather than using negative energy, we have found that the best motivator for healthful change is *self-love*. To embrace a healthy lifestyle, you must see yourself as valuable and worth "fixing." Each time you nourish your body with healthy foods, meditate to a state of emotional serenity, or stretch and use your muscles in sports or exercise, you are affirming yourself. In addition, your health-affirming behaviors allow you to serve as a living example of positive health to your coworkers, family, friends, and neighbors. As African Americans, we can change our health profile, but we must do it one person at a time.

LEARNING TO TRUST

It's a classic self-fulfilling prophecy: People who suspect that they are sick refuse to seek medical care when they first detect a medical problem because they worry that the doctor will confirm their fears. Then, when they finally get around to contacting a doctor, their fears are realized: Their conditions have progressed to the point that their prognosis is much worse. Regrettably, this pattern of delayed care and poor prognosis is classic in the African American community.

One patient who illustrates the point quite well is a woman who came into the office complaining of pain and abdominal distension. She did not contact a doctor until the pain was unbearable and she had no other choice. Upon examination, we learned that she suffered from a rectal mass so large that it had totally blocked her bowel function. If she had been treated earlier, we probably could have saved her life, but since she came to us after the cancer had spread, there was little we could do. When asked why she had taken so long to see a doctor, she said, "The hospital is where you go to die, and I am not ready to die yet." Both her sister and her mother had died in the hospital, and she had a strong association between hospital care and death. Ironically, her fear and distrust of the medical establishment is what ultimately killed her.

We have found that a lot of patients have the same reaction to treatment for HIV and AIDS. Many African Americans who live in the inner city have friends who have taken the drug AZT and newer medications as part of their treatment for the disease, only to see them die a few months later. It was not the AZT or other medication that killed the patient, but rather the deadly delay in seeking help. Of course, if they had taken the drug and received treatment earlier, many lives would have been extended. These stories and others like them create a distorted perception about what medical science can do. Unfortunately, such scenarios are all too common in our community.

This distrust of Western medicine is one of the reasons for the bad health statistics for African Americans. We must learn to overcome our fears and take charge of our health; we should start by getting accurate and complete information about our health.

One of the biggest problems is denial: Denial will not make us well. Denial will not help the man with chest pains who doesn't want to go to the hospital when he knows good and well that he is experiencing a heart attack. Denial won't help the woman who refuses to take an HIV test because she suspects she is HIV positive.

While some of us may have a fear of dealing with the medical establishment, we must take responsibility for our health care. That may mean finding a medical doctor who is informed and sensitive to the unique health needs of African American patients, and it may mean consulting with practitioners of natural medicine who can offer a complementary approach to healing. Keep in mind, however, that both conventional and complementary healers cannot make you well if they do not know that you are sick.

BEING GENTLE WITH OURSELVES

If you are challenged with fears or resist taking steps to care for yourself, that's okay. You should simply start with small steps. The key to moving in this direction is to just start moving. Begin with something you know you can do, then build on that. The key is to be gentle with yourself while you are learning to honor and nurture yourself.

If you run into your own resistance along the way, use some of the following affirmations to inspire you. Write them out and put them in a place where you can see them during the day. Changing a habit takes time, so be patient with yourself. After working with thousands of people, we know that you can make positive changes for yourself.

Start with these affirmations (or write one of your own). Read your favorite one every day for a week, then switch to another:

- I am worthy of my own attention.

- It is okay for me to take care of myself as well as others.

- Doing for myself, I am learning how to really care for others.

- How many times I fall down doesn't matter. The fact that I get back up is what counts.

- God don't make no junk. The fact that I am here means that I am somebody.

- When I take care of myself and love myself, I start to see the meaning of who I am.

THESE TESTS CAN SAVE YOUR LIFE

One of the best ways to take care of ourselves—and to catch illnesses at the early stages—is to undergo routine medical screening tests. These procedures, while sometimes uncomfortable or bothersome, do save lives. It's always heartbreaking to receive a diagnosis of a serious illness, but it is particularly distressing when the problem could have been controlled or reversed if only it had been caught at an earlier stage.

While natural remedies can be helpful in the treatment and management of disease, you must know you have a health problem before you can treat it. We recommend the following screening tests.

SCREENING TESTS AND EXAMS FOR AFRICAN AMERICANS

These tests should be routinely performed; others may be necessary if recommended by your physician or if your medical history dictates:

- **Blood pressure measurement.** Annually after age fifty; more often if under treatment for hypertension. Blood pressure is taken as part of a routine physical exam. Between physicals, you may want to test your blood pressure yourself. Many pharmacies and grocery stores have machines available for public use; stop in twice a year and have your blood pressure checked.

- **Breast exam** (women). Monthly at home; annually by your doctor.

- **Cholesterol.** Begin testing at adolescence. Test every five years, or more often if you have a history of atherosclerosis or coronary disease. You should look for both your total cholesterol levels as well as your high-density lipoprotein (HDL) and low-density lipoprotein (LDL) levels. (For more information on cholesterol and for target levels, see Chapter 12, "Mending Our Hearts," page 213.)

- **Complete physical.** Every five years before age forty; every two years between ages forty and sixty, and annually thereafter.

- **Dental exam and tooth cleaning.** Every six months; more often if periodontal disease is present.

- **Dental X rays.** Every one to two years.

- **Electrocardiogram.** Every three years after age forty; more often if there is evidence of heart disease.

- **Eye examination.** Every one to two years.

- **Mammography** (women). Every one to two years between ages forty and forty-nine; annually age fifty and older. If you have a family history of breast cancer, a mammogram may be recommended even earlier.

- **Occult blood in stool.** Annually after age forty.

- **Pelvic exam** (women). Annually, including a Pap smear and digital rectal exam.

- **Prostate exam** (men). Annually at age forty and above; annually after age thirty-five if there is a family history of the disease. We rely on both a physical exam and the prostate-specific antigen test, which can detect prostate cancer early. The PSA test can provide helpful information, but it is not a substitute for a physical exam.

- **Rectal exam/digital.** Annually after age thirty-five.

- **Sigmoidoscopy.** Every three to five years after age forty.

- **Skin exam.** Once a month, using a mirror or asking a friend for help, check every square inch of your skin for abnormalities, including moles, rashes, or scaling. Annually, have a primary care physician or dermatologist perform a skin check, starting at age forty, or earlier if you have a lot of sun-related skin damage.

- **Testicular exam** (men). This should be done as part of a physical. Monthly self-exams are highly recommended. (An ideal time is when you are in the shower.)

▼▼▼▼▼▼▼▼▼▼▼▼▼▼▼▼▼▼▼▼▼▼▼▼▼▼▼

FOR MORE INFORMATION

For general information on disease prevention and treatment for African Americans, contact the Office of Minority Health Resource

Center, P.O. Box 37337, Washington, DC 20013-7337; (800) 444-6472 or (301) 587-1938. The Internet address is http://www.omhrc.gov. The resource center operates a library, provides written materials, offers referrals, and answers questions regarding minority health issues.

▲▲▲▲▲▲▲▲▲▲▲▲▲▲▲▲▲▲▲▲▲▲▲▲▲▲▲▲▲▲▲

2
▼

East Meets West

Understanding the Natural Approach to Wellness

*Balance is essential to health, and imbalance
creates, or is, disease.*
HIPPOCRATES

Many of the patients who come into our offices are skeptics. They want to believe in Western medicine, but they feel it has let them down. They want to believe in natural healing, but it is unfamiliar. Consider the case of a sixty-two-year-old retired concert pianist and professor who was referred to the practice by a relative. This patient kept meticulous records about his blood pressure medications; he took them like clockwork. When we talked about trading in some of his blood pressure medications for herbs and supplements, a look of concern crossed his face. "I feel fine, so why rock the boat?" he asked. His blood pressure was 158/90 most of the time, and he was not interested in playing games.

We started treatment slowly, but over time he began to feel more confident about the natural approach. He realized that his blood pressure could be lower and he decided to try new treatments. Gradually, we added a few supplements and cut down on his medications. His blood pressure dropped to the lowest level it had been since he developed hypertension, and he takes less than half the medications he did when he first came to the office. He now believes in natural healing, and he may soon be off all of his blood pressure medication and on only natural nutritional supplements.

The truth is that modern medicine really can deliver miracles. A heart damaged by atherosclerosis can be rebuilt during bypass surgery; a diabetic pancreas that can no longer pump insulin can be supplanted by regular insulin injections; lenses clouded by cataracts can be surgically replaced with plastic lenses. While such man-made miracles offer great promise in many situations, there are other times that natural remedies can offer greater hope than conventional medicine.

In recent years, a growing number of Americans of every race have rediscovered the benefits of natural medicine. Disillusioned with the invasiveness—and often the ineffectiveness—of many conventional treatments, many open-minded people have turned to practitioners of natural medicine for help. The limitations of conventional medicine have lead to a greater acceptance of alternative approaches to healing. We predict that the African American community will lead the way in the health care revolution because it represents a return to our native roots of healing. African Americans have been denied access to conventional health care for most of our history, but we have been able to draw on a rich tradition of folk medicine and family remedies. For many of us, those homespun healing techniques included the use of herbs and nutrition—as well as the recuperative powers of the mind and spirit.

Natural medicine is based on the simple but profound belief that the human body has an amazing ability to heal itself. The practitioner's role is to assist the body in the healing process, not simply to suppress the symptoms of disease. As part of this philosophy, we must view the body holistically: We must focus on the overall condition of the patient, not just the part that is injured or sick. Conventional physicians tend to deal with the symptoms of disease rather than the root cause. The major focus is to suppress the symptom or complaint, rather than to strengthen the system.

You don't have to choose between conventional medicine and natural medicine; instead, you can borrow the best of both approaches to healing and customize them to your particular situation. We believe that natural medicine should be used as the first course of treatment or as an adjunct to conventional medicine. Of course, let both your conventional physician and practitioner of natural medicine know about the treatment provided by the other. In some cases, the treatments may conflict with one another; for example, an herbal remedy might react with or diminish the effectiveness of a prescribed drug, or vice versa. In the end, a cooperative approach that includes both traditional treatments and natural remedies will probably provide the best care for your overall health.

THE ENERGETIC BODY

The cornerstone of natural medicine is the understanding of the body's energy system. We all intuitively know that this system exists. As physicians, we have lost track of the number of times when asked, "How are you doing?" our patients have responded, "I am out of energy." We can all feel the energy reserves in our bodies and we know when our energy system is out of balance.

Practitioners of Chinese medicine have known about the energetic body for more than two thousand years. Chinese healers refer to the concept of *qi* and describe how this energy circulates around the body. Instead of studying this energy as an abstract life force, Western scientists have studied it as bioelectrical impulses that light up the human body.

One of the first things we learned in medical school was that each cell in the human body contains a pump that works very hard at keeping potassium inside the cell and sodium outside the cell. This electrolyte balance keeps an electrical charge going across the cell membrane. We also learned that nerves in the body send electrical impulses, which can be turned into chemical messages that affect the way our organs do their jobs. In a memorable lesson, we also learned that the heart transmits an electrical wave of energy with every beat. We are all electrically charged; we are the body electric.

Albert Szent-Gyorgyi (who had already won a Nobel Prize for his work on oxidation and vitamin C) first suggested the concept of a larger energy system of the human body more than half a century ago. He argued that in order to fully understand the human body and biochemistry, scientists needed to look into an energy system that runs throughout the body. "It looks as if we are missing some basic fact about life, without which any real understanding is impossible," he said. He went on to theorize that human cells are structured in such a way that they perfectly conduct energy, much like a semiconductor that can transmit low-energy impulses over long distances. This is the same type of energy system that is found in computers and satellites.

Robert O. Becker, M.D., and others have further studied this concept and found that the human body includes a very organized network of electrical charges. Energy vitalizes our cells; if we lose this charge, we die. Researchers have also showed that the electrical charge of the human body is very specific. The brain and spine tend to be positively charged, and the hands, feet, and front of the body are negatively charged.

Like many other practitioners of natural medicine, we believe that many health problems begin with an imbalance in the energetic system. In many cases, this system falls out of balance months or years before health problems show up on blood tests, X rays, and other conventional tests. Our experiences with our patients support the findings of European researchers who have found that up to 70 percent of the problems that are seen in a primary care physician's office stem from energetic imbalances. This may help explain why so many patients complain of health problems, even though the blood work and results of other medical tests are normal. These people are told, "The doctor can't find anything wrong," but the doctor may not understand that the problem stems from an energetic disturbance.

To illustrate this point with our patients, we often remind them that many people with arthritis can tell when it's going to rain before there is a cloud in the sky. Eventually the clouds form, turn dark, and the rain falls. Clearly, the body has an early warning system that alerts the person to the change in weather.

The same thing happens when there is an imbalance of the body's energy system. If the body is out of balance energetically for a long period of time, the energy eventually stops circulating through the body normally. This then throws off the functions of the organs of the body and leads to disease. At this point, we can begin to see the health problems show up in the various tests that we do in Western medicine. In our medical practices, we try to use natural medicine to balance the energetic imbalances before the problem reaches this point.

THE BODY IN HARMONY

The body's energy system transmits information along special energy circuits or pathways between the cells, between muscles and tendons, and outside the blood vessels and nerves. As it travels along these pathways, named *meridians* by the ancient Chinese, the energy vibrates at a given pitch in a given energy channel. The key to healing the body is keeping these energy channels well tuned with the proper nutrition, supplements, and stimulation. When the energy channels are out of balance, the body falls out of harmony, leading to disease.

The meridians are active in a newborn baby, and they continue to function throughout our lives. You can use a number of techniques to keep these channels open. Simple walking helps stretch and flex the arms and legs to open the channels. Massage, acupressure, and therapeutic touch work in the same way.

In addition, many natural remedies attempt to alter the vibration of the energy channels. Anything that is alive has an energy field. Since herbs and many homeopathic remedies come from living plants, they retain the energy fingerprint of the plant. In other words, the fingerprint that is left is the harmonic pitch, or vibration rate, which is unique for any given plant or supplement. These herbs and homeopathic supplements can clear these channels because they have an energy signature that can restore the vibration of a human body that is out of pitch in a given channel. (For more information on energetics, see Chapter 3, "Mind, Body, Spirit, Soul," page 41.)

A BRIEF INTRODUCTION TO FOUR KEY TECHNIQUES

As physicians and natural healers, we use literally dozens of techniques in the treatment of our patients. However, most of the advice we offer in this book will focus on four common types of natural medicine: herbal medicine, nutritional supplements, homeopathy, and acupuncture and acupressure. Of course, not every technique can be used for every medical problem, but we have tried to include a range of treatment options in the hope that one will meet your needs and interests.

Herbal Medicine

In some African American families, knowledge of herbal medicine is passed from generation to generation as part of an informal but highly effective system of folk health care. As a result of this exposure to the use of herbs, many of our African American patients feel quite comfortable using herbs "just like my grandmother used to do."

Nature offers almost everything you need to stock your medicine cabinet. Herbal remedies (or botanicals) can be used to treat most common conditions and ailments. They are often safer, cheaper, and more effective than synthetic drugs, and they can be used to treat a handful of conditions that mainstream medicines can't touch, such as viral infections like influenza. That's not to say that man-made drugs have no place in your medicine cabinet. However, in many cases, herbal medicine can be used to treat problems before they get to the stage where conventional medicine is needed.

In Africa our ancestors relied on the natural healing ability of plants to treat almost every ailment, from conditions associated with infancy to those of old age. Today, four out of five people worldwide use herbs as the basis of their medical care. Though most Americans rely on synthetic drugs produced in a laboratory, European doctors often prescribe herbal treatments for their patients. In fact, half of the prescriptions German doctors write for depression are for Saint-John's-wort, an herb, rather than for man-made psychoactive drugs.

One of the main reasons that synthetic medicines are more popular than herbs in the United States is that drug companies can patent those drugs they create, but they cannot patent Mother Nature's cures. Still, about 70 percent of all prescription drugs sold in the United States contain active ingredients isolated from plants, and most synthetic drugs are little more than synthesized versions of chemicals that occur naturally in plants. Consider digitalis, a prescription drug used in the treatment of congestive heart failure and arrhythmia. This chemical is derived from the plant foxglove, which is grown in Holland. Painkillers such as morphine or codeine are derived from the opium poppy; the cancer drugs vincristine and vinblastine come from periwinkle; and even old-fashioned aspirin finds its origins with the salicin in willow bark.

Herbal medicines are better balanced and buffered than their man-made counterparts. Plants bring an energetic quality to the treatment that is missing from synthetic medicines. While pharmacists have been able to isolate certain active ingredients in herbs, a plant actually contains hundreds of agents that work together. The synergy between the natural ingredients helps explain why whole plants tend to be more effective—with fewer negative side effects—than single-ingredient remedies. Man can't produce a cure that is as balanced and complete as Nature can.

▼▼▼▼▼▼▼▼▼▼▼▼▼▼▼▼▼▼▼▼▼▼▼▼▼▼▼

OUR HERITAGE OF HEALING

Our African ancestors were among the first healers to use herbs as medicines, perhaps as much as ten thousand years ago. At that time, medicinal knowledge was taught to monks in monasteries or temples. In time, these monks, who could also be called herbalists, shared their knowledge with European healers, who adopted the methods for European culture. So, while many people assume that herbal healing has its roots in Europe, it can actually be traced back to African empires such as Mali, Songhi, and Kush.

▲▲▲▲▲▲▲▲▲▲▲▲▲▲▲▲▲▲▲▲▲▲▲▲▲▲▲

Strong Medicine

Many people who agonize over taking an over-the-counter painkiller think nothing of swallowing an herbal treatment because they consider it "natural" and therefore not dangerous. Herbs that have the ability to heal also have the ability to harm if misused. Yes, in general herbal remedies are safer and have fewer side effects than man-made drugs, but they can have potent and harmful side effects, and they should be treated with the same respect. Like any other drugs, herbs can have negative—and sometimes dangerous—side effects if taken in excessive doses.

Part of the confusion about safety stems from the way herbal treatments are labeled. Unlike synthetic drugs, herbal remedies do not have to go through the formal approval process from the U.S. Food and Drug Administration because they are classified as foods or food additives rather than drugs. This means that manufacturers of herbal remedies must be cautious about the claims they make on package labels—drug-related claims and warnings are prohibited. Consumers must be on their toes about understanding the products they are buying. Read the package directions carefully, and always follow the dosage information on the product label. If you have any questions about how a product should be used, do not use it until you contact the product manufacturer, a qualified herbalist, or a professional organization dedicated to the safe use of herbs for more information. (For a list of resources on herbs, see page 315.)

You can find many herbal remedies in health food stores, but recently they have begun showing up in conventional supermarkets and pharmacies as well. If you can't find what you need at local stores, refer to the listing on page 317 for information on mail-order companies that sell herbs.

Most of the herbal treatments listed in this book involve single herbs rather than formulas, blends of herbs designed to act synergistically to achieve specific results for a specific individual. Ideally, a formula is prepared for the specific needs of an individual patient, but packaged formulas often work quite well and they are readily available at health food stores. In this book, we refer to individual herbs in the remedies we recommend only because mixing formulas requires the expertise of a professional.

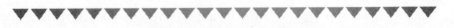

Our History of Healing

Female African slaves brought herbs to many countries by braiding seeds into the cornrows in their hair. As a result, in many places where African slaves are found, so are the herbs used in African herbal healing.

Using Herbs

While all herbal medicines use plant material, different medicines employ different parts of the plant, such as the leaves, seeds, flowers, roots, bark, or berries. The particular "recipes" for herbal remedies have been refined and improved by herbalists over thousands of years. Though only a tiny fraction of the world's plants have been tested for their medicinal potential, American herbalists use approximately one thousand different herbs to treat everything from Alzheimer's disease to varicose veins.

We recommend commercial herbal preparations for most of our patients, but some people prefer to prepare their remedies themselves, using whole plants. Whether purchased at a health food store or prepared in a home kitchen, herbal medicines come in one of several forms (listed in increasing order of potency):

- **Teas.** Made by steeping about 1 teaspoon of dried herbs or 3 teaspoons of fresh herbs in 1 cup of boiling water for 5 minutes or so, then straining. Most herbal teas are not strong enough to provide medicinal value.

- **Infusions.** Made much the same way as strong tea, with several important differences. The water should be just short of boiling (since boiling water disperses important volatile oils in the steam), and the herbs are steeped for 20 to 30 minutes, so the resulting liquid is much more potent and often more bitter. The infusion should be strained before drinking. Most infusions are made with ½ to 1 rounded teaspoon of dried herbs or 3 teaspoons of fresh herbs per cup of water. The standard dose is ½ cup three times a day.

- **Decoctions.** Made like infusions, only the bark, roots, or berries of the herbs are simmered (never boiled), rather than merely steeped, for 20 to 30 minutes (or sometimes longer). Most decoctions are made with ½ to 1 rounded teaspoon of dried herbs per cup of water. The standard dose is ½ cup three times a day.

- **Tinctures.** Made by soaking herbs in an alcohol solution (25 percent alcohol/75 percent water) for a specified period of time (from several hours to several days, depending on the herb). Commercial tinctures use ethyl alcohol, but apple cider vinegar, vodka, brandy, and rum are suitable for home use (and the brandy and rum can help to disguise the bitter flavor of some herbs). Because alcohol acts as a preservative, tinctures can be stored for up to two years. Use 1 ounce of crushed dried herbs with 5 ounces of alcohol solution (1.25 ounces alcohol/3.75 ounces water) for 6 weeks. When preparing a tincture, shake the mixture every few days to encourage alcohol uptake of the herb's active ingredients. WARNING: Do not use methyl alcohol or isopropyl alcohol (rubbing alcohol) when making tinctures; they are toxic if taken internally.

- **Extracts.** Made by distilling some of the alcohol off of a tincture, leaving a more potent concentrate behind. Most commercial extracts use vacuum distillation or filtration techniques, which do not require the use of high temperatures.

- **Powdered herbs.** Made by removing the moisture from an extract, then grinding the solid herbal concentrate into granules or powders, which can be shaped into capsules or tablets. We prefer the use of capsules over tablets because some of the active ingredients are destroyed when the powder is squeezed (at a pressure of more than 400 pounds per square inch) to form the tablet.

Sometimes infusions or decoctions have a sharp, bitter taste. You need to be aware of this when using these blends. Part of the therapy has to do with the taste; by stimulating certain taste buds, the treatment begins before it hits your stomach. You can also purchase prepared tinctures, extracts, or powdered herbs and follow the dosage information on the product labels.

Herbal mixtures or blends of herbs work best when the ingredients balance one another. When a treatment is properly balanced, the side effects should be rare. However, before using herbs, check with your doctor, since herbal medicines can interact with conventional drugs. Use only the recommended amounts and take herbs only for the recommended time periods. The risk of side effects goes up when people take large amounts of herbs for extended periods.

Watch out for symptoms of overdose or toxicity. Typical symptoms include stomach upset, nausea, diarrhea, or headache an hour or two after taking an herb. If you develop any of these signs of overdose after taking an herb, stop taking it and see if the symptoms disappear. If you experience a negative side effect associated with an herb, contact your health care practitioner and report it to the FDA's MedWatch office at (800) 332-1088.

Diet and Nutritional Supplements

Even under the best of circumstances, it is very difficult to get all the vitamins and minerals you need from the foods you eat. At the turn of the century, crops were grown in fields with forty inches of mineral-rich topsoil; today it is estimated that there is less than four inches of topsoil in many fields, severely limiting the mineral content in many vegetables and fruits. In addition, African Americans face special challenges because they often eat a poorly balanced diet and prepare foods in ways that deplete the nutritional value.

Taking daily nutritional and mineral supplements can make up for many shortcomings in your diet. Studies have found that people who took a daily multiple vitamin supplement had stronger immune systems and suffered fewer infections than those who did not take the supplements. Supplements can also be used to treat disease once it has taken hold. The specific, prescriptive advice offered later in the book explains how supplements can be used in the treatment of a number of ailments and conditions. For more information, see Chapter 9, "Enough Is Not Always Enough: Using Nutritional Supplements," page 149.

Homeopathy

Homeopathy is based on the premise that less is more. This holistic approach to healing relies on the use of infinitesimal amounts of substances—plants, minerals, chemicals, microorganisms, animal materials, and even modern drugs—to boost the body's defenses against illness. Homeopathy can be a very effective tool in the treatment of colds, headaches, and many other problems.

One of the principal tenets of homeopathy is the Law of Similars—

or "like cures like"—a theory that a remedy taken in small amounts will cure the same symptoms that it would cause if taken in large amounts. In fact, the word *homeopathy* has its roots in the Greek words *homo,* meaning "like, similar," and *pathos,* meaning "suffering or disease."

Consider the medicinal use of belladonna, an extract from the poisonous plant deadly nightshade. If taken internally, belladonna can cause high fever, flushed face, confusion, and other flulike symptoms. However, belladonna is one of the homeopathic remedies for fever and flu precisely because it causes these symptoms. Of course, the actual amount of belladonna used in the homeopathic remedy is dramatically diluted. In fact, the active ingredients in homeopathic remedies are diluted to such a degree that not a single molecule of the active ingredients can be found in the solution in its final form. Despite the dilution, there is evidence that homeopathic remedies work, as you will see later in this chapter.

The dependence on dilution illustrates the second law of homeopathy, the Law of Infinitesimals. This theory states that the smaller the dose of an active ingredient, the more effective the cure. However, for this less-is-more principle to work, each time the solution is diluted it must be "potentized" (or shaken) to create "memory of the energy" that cures the body. The Law of Infinitesimals was discovered through careful experimentation by Dr. Samuel Christian Hahnemann (1755–1843), the founder of the practice of homeopathy.

Putting Homeopathy to the Test

Even the staunchest supporters of homeopathy must admit that the theories of homeopathy defy many of the laws of physical science as we know them. Skeptics charge that any healing that takes places stems from the placebo effect (the benefit a patient gets just by believing that a particular treatment will work). However, a number of studies published in respected medical journals have shown that homeopathic remedies work. Consider the evidence:

- 1986: Researchers in Scotland gave a homeopathic hay fever remedy to 144 people with a pollen allergy. To eliminate prejudice on the part of the researchers, the study was double-blind and placebo-controlled, meaning neither the researchers nor the participants knew who was receiving the homeopathic remedy and who was receiving the placebo. Compared with those who took the placebo, the homeopathic group showed a significant reduction in symptoms, and their need for antihistamines dropped by 50 percent.

- 1989: Nonhomeopathic researchers in Great Britain conducted a double-blind, placebo-controlled study to test a homeopathic flu remedy on nearly five hundred people. After two days the homeopathic remedy relieved twice as many flu symptoms as the placebo.

- 1990: German researchers tested eight homeopathic remedies on sixty-one people with varicose veins as part of a double-blind, placebo-controlled study. Among the participants who took the homeopathic remedies, symptoms improved by 44 percent; among those who took the placebo, symptoms became 18 percent worse.

- 1991: *The British Medical Journal* published an analysis of 105 clinical studies involving the efficacy of homeopathy. The homeopathic treatment was found to be more effective than a placebo in eighty-one of the studies. Critics of homeopathy charged that many of the studies were poorly designed, but a review of twenty-six of the better controlled studies found that fifteen demonstrated the benefit of homeopathic treatments.

- 1994: A study published in the British medical journal *The Lancet* found that homeopathic treatments outperformed a placebo in bringing relief to twenty-eight patients allergic to dust mites.

- 1994: The peer-reviewed American medical journal *Pediatrics* reported that among eighty-one children in Nicaragua treated for diarrhea, those given a homeopathic treatment in addition to the standard oral rehydration therapy got well faster than those who got the standard treatment alone. Among the children in the control group, the diarrhea lasted an average of four days, but in the group receiving the homeopathic treatment, it lasted 2½ days.

Despite the mounting evidence, no one really understands exactly how or why homeopathy works. Some researchers have speculated that the "potentization"—the repeated diluting and shaking of the substances—creates a distinctive electrochemical pattern in the water. According to this theory of energy medicine, when a patient takes the homeopathic remedy, the electrochemical pattern in the solution somehow subtly changes the electromagnetic fields in the body. We believe that this is the mechanism that makes homeopathy effective. The correct homeopathic product creates a vibration in your system; it sets up a harmonic pitch in your meridian channels. Your body remembers that tone, and starts to harmonize and sing along with it.

Not all scientists accept this explanation, and ultimately the question of how homeopathy works remains open. But you can take advantage of the healing benefits of homeopathy without understanding all of its mysteries. All you need to do is keep an open mind and learn more about how you can use homeopathy to manage a number of illnesses and ailments.

Practicing Homeopathy

A visit to a homeopath is nothing like a visit to a conventional physician. Homeopaths and medical doctors approach healing from different points of view. Homeopaths treat the person, not the disease. They believe that illness is not localized in one organ or manifested in a single symptom. When deciding which of the three thousand homeopathic remedies they should prescribe for a patient, they consider the entire person, both mind and body.

In contrast, conventional physicians typically focus on suppressing symptoms, taking little or no account of the person's emotional or overall physical condition. They see their mission as one of lowering fevers, easing aches and pains, and eliminating other symptoms or complaints, rather than treating the person as a whole.

These marked differences in approach show up in the first office visit. While a conventional doctor might spend less than ten minutes with a patient, a homeopath can spend over an hour interviewing that patient, asking detailed questions about medical history and personal characteristics. The homeopath will construct a patient profile based on overall energy, sensitivity to temperature, sleep habits, food preferences, emotional state, and other factors that help the homeopath understand the patient and prescribe the best remedy for the individual.

Unlike this customized system of medicine, the selection of the appropriate homeopathic remedy varies from patient to patient, depending on the patient's individual needs, rather than the symptoms. For example, two people might pass a cold virus from one to the other, but each person would receive different treatments, based on his or her specific personal needs.

Despite its many benefits, homeopathy is not the best treatment for all illnesses or conditions. It is not appropriate for medical problems that involve physical deformities, tissue damage, cancer, or for situations that might require surgery. Since it can take a great deal of experience and expertise to determine which homeopathic remedies would work best in a given situation, the remedies outlined in Part 3 of this book tend to be general. You should limit your home use of homeopathic remedies to treatment of relatively minor or straightforward ailments. If you try a remedy and fail to find relief, consult a trained homeopath.

Finding the Right Solution

To ensure efficacy and purity, homeopathic remedies are prepared according to the standards of the *Homeopathic Pharmacopoeia of the United States*. First, the raw material or active ingredient is dissolved in an alcohol/water mixture that contains about 90 percent pure alcohol and 10 percent distilled water. The mixture then stands for two to four weeks, with periodic shakings. It is then strained, and the resulting liquid is known as the mother tincture.

Homeopathic remedies come in a variety of potencies, based on the number of times they were diluted. Topical homeopathic creams, ointments, and salves can be made by mixing the tincture with a cream or gel base. The three most common forms of homeopathic remedies are the mother tincture, x potencies, and c potencies.

The mother tincture. The mother tincture is an alcohol-based extract of a specific substance. Mother tinctures are usually used topically.

X potencies. The x represents the Roman numeral 10. In homeopathic remedies with x potencies the mother tincture has been diluted to one part in ten (one drop of tincture to every nine drops of alcohol/

water solution). The number before the x tells how many times the mother tincture has been diluted. For example, a 12x potency represents 12 dilutions of one in ten. The more the substance is diluted, the more potent it becomes, so a remedy with a 30x potency is considered stronger or more potent than one with a 12x potency. The more you dilute it, the stronger it gets.

C potencies. The c represents the Roman numeral 100. Homeopathic remedies with a c potency have been diluted to one part in 100 (one drop of tincture to every 99 drops of alcohol/water solution). Again, the number before the c represents the number of dilutions. By the time 3c is reached, the dilution is one part per million. In most cases, 6c is the potency recommended for acute or self-limiting ailments, and 30c for chronic conditions or emergencies.

The 30c potency should not be administered for more than four doses without a clear and definite result. If your condition improves after four doses, wait and see what happens. If the symptoms return, take up to four more doses, then wait again. If you experience no improvement after four doses, discontinue the treatment and try something else or contact a qualified homeopath.

Homocords. This is a liquid preparation that has several strengths mixed together. In this preparation, your body picks the strength (or pitch) that it needs to help it regain function.

Homeopathic remedies come in pellet, tablet, and liquid forms. The pellets and tablets consist primarily of sugar (they actually contain milk sugar, or lactose, so people with lactose intolerance should use a liquid form). When taking homeopathic pellets or tablets, avoid touching them. Instead, shake the pellets into a measuring spoon and place them in your mouth to allow them to dissolve. Unless otherwise noted, a dose is one tablet, one drop, or just enough pellets to cover the area of the small fingernail.

When taking a homeopathic remedy, do not eat for at least a half hour before or after taking it. Strong flavors can decrease the effectiveness of the remedies. Likewise, avoid strong odors, which can also affect the efficacy of the treatment.

If you are using an appropriate homeopathic remedy, it should work quickly, and then you can discontinue treatment. Although negative reactions to homeopathic remedies are rare, they can happen. If your condition gets worse after taking a particular remedy, stop taking it. Wait for the aggravation to subside and then try it again. If the problems resurface, stop using the remedy and seek help from a professional homeopath.

Homeopathic remedies will not interfere with any drugs your doctor prescribes for you. However, many conventional drugs—including steroids, tranquilizers, oral contraceptives, sleeping pills, and antihistamines—can modify or completely block the effects of homeopathic drugs. Discuss any drug reactions with your doctor. Do not stop taking any drugs—especially prescription drugs—without first consulting your doctor.

Acupuncture and Acupressure

A generation ago, Americans learned what the Chinese have known for more than five thousand years: Through the practice of acupressure we can stimulate the body's natural ability to heal itself.

The ancient healing arts of acupressure and acupuncture involve the use of either fingertip pressure or fine needles to activate a network of key pressure points, promoting muscle relaxation and increasing blood circulation. Healers have refined the techniques over the centuries as they have observed and recorded the relationships between healing and touch at various points on the body.

Acupressurists and acupuncturists use two types of pressure points: trigger points (pressure points located where the pain occurs) and acupressure points (pressure points located far from the site where the pain occurs). Acupressure points stimulate a response in distant parts of the body because they lie along a network of energy channels (called meridians) that run throughout the body. Ancient Chinese healers have identified twelve major meridians, each named after or corresponding to a different organ, such as large intestine, small intestine, or bladder.

The meridians connect the acupressure points in what can be considered an invisible wiring system for the flow of bioelectrical impulses, or the body's "essential life energy," known as *chi* or *qi* in Chinese. Traditional Chinese healers believe that chi comes in two opposite but complementary forms, yin (passive energy) and yang (active energy). When these two types of chi are balanced, the body is in harmony and in good health. When someone suffers from an injury or illness, however, chi falls out of balance. To correct an imbalance, you need to stimulate one or more of the appropriate pressure points.

Western healers may not accept the traditional explanation for how acupressure works, but researchers are collecting evidence showing that it does. Research shows that acupressure stimulates the release of endorphins, the body's natural painkillers and mood and immune-system regulators. In fact, studies have shown that endorphin levels in the brain double thirty minutes after a session of acupuncture.

Skeptics have argued that the benefits attributed to acupressure and acupuncture should be attributed instead to the placebo effect, or the ability of a patient's expectations to influence his or her reported experience of healing. However, studies have shown that acupuncture proves effective in pain control 55 to 85 percent of the time, much more than can be explained by the placebo effect alone.

While not intended to replace conventional medical care, acupuncture (in the hands of a trained professional) or acupressure (as a method of self-care) may help you manage illness and control pain in many situations. As thousands of years of experience has proved, when used properly, these techniques can be safe and effective in treating many illnesses.

Getting to the Point

To the beginner, acupressure can seem complex and intimidating. But once you begin to experiment with the technique, it will become very natural, and you will be able to enjoy its relaxing and healing benefits.

To help you find the point—or, more precisely, each of the body's 365 named and numbered acupressure points—experts have developed elaborate maps of the human body, using joints, muscles, and indentations in the bones as physical landmarks. The body is symmetrical, and most acupressure points are bilateral, occurring on both sides of the body. Except when an acupressure point falls on the midline of the body, acupressure should be applied to points on both sides.

When practicing acupressure, you'll know you've found the correct point (also known as *tsubo*) if the person who is being treated feels a tingle, "charge," or electrical impulse when you apply direct pressure; the point may also feel tender. In most cases, these points are located along the bones or beneath the major muscle groups. If the point is tender, your body is telling you it needs treatment. Over time, that point should become less sensitive.

After locating the correct spot, you will use your thumbs, middle fingers, palms, or the side of your hands to apply firm, steady pressure. Your finger should be held at a right angle to the body. Start with a gentle touch and gradually push harder until you feel a deep, even pressure, but not pain. Remember that fleshy parts of the body can withstand firmer pressure than bony areas. During an acupressure session, work the points on both sides of the body to maintain balance and harmony in your body.

Three to five minutes of steady, firm pressure works best, but as little as one minute can begin to promote healing and quiet the nervous system. At the end of an acupressure session, you should feel relaxed and invigorated, but don't expect that the pain will subside and your symptoms will disappear immediately. Acupressure isn't a matter of pressing a button and exacting a "cure"; long-term results require regular practice. It often takes at least four to six months of regular practice to see substantial pain relief for prolonged periods of time, so be patient. For the best results, plan on spending fifteen minutes or so working through your acupressure points two or three times a day, if you can. But whatever you can do will be helpful.

Hints for Hands-on Healing

- Before starting your acupressure session, take a few minutes to relax and get focused. If possible, settle into a quiet, warm, and well-ventilated room. Start with some deep breathing to help you relax (see page 69). During your session, try to focus your thoughts on the healing process and visualize the pain or illness disappearing.

- If you are practicing acupressure on yourself, some points will be difficult to press without straining. To reach points on your back, place a soft tennis ball on a carpet and smoothly roll over onto it while supporting most of your weight on your elbows. If this is impossible to do without discomfort, either skip the point or recruit a friend to help.

- Keep your fingernails short to avoid scratching or poking your skin.

- Make sure to smoothly and gradually increase the pressure, and smoothly and gradually release the pressure. Avoid sharp pokes or jabs.

- Remember that acupressure should not hurt. If a point feels painful to the touch, work on it more gently or gradually release the pressure and move to another point.

- Avoid contact with areas that have been burned, bruised, cut, sprained, or infected. If the surrounding area is not too tender, consider applying pressure to the points near the injury to stimulate blood flow and to promote healing in the area.

- If you feel particularly stiff or tense before a session, consider soaking in a hot bath or applying a hot-water bottle or heating pad to the affected area before beginning treatment. Adding slices of ginger-root to the bathwater can help the soothing heat reach into the muscles and energy channels. (This is especially helpful in the cold winter months.)

- If possible, wait at least an hour after eating before practicing acupressure. Also avoid scheduling your acupressure sessions during times when you feel particularly hungry.

▼▼▼▼▼▼▼▼▼▼▼▼▼▼▼▼▼▼▼▼▼▼▼▼

DR. WALKER: PUTTING ACUPUNCTURE TO THE TEST

In my practice I strive to build bridges between Eastern and Western medicine. In 1997 I was able to help reinforce that connection by participating in an expert panel convened by the National Institutes of Health to evaluate the scientific merits of acupuncture. During the 2½-day consensus conference, dozens of scientists with differing backgrounds and points of view reviewed clinical studies and debated the risks and benefits of acupuncture.

In the end, we found clear evidence that acupuncture is safe and effective for a range of medical conditions, including pain following dental surgery and nausea associated with chemotherapy, pregnancy, and surgery. The panel concluded that acupuncture can also be helpful in the treatment of headache, low back pain, carpal tunnel syndrome, stroke, menstrual cramps, asthma, and addiction, among other problems. Since conventional treatment is limited, the panel felt that acupuncture was a reasonable treatment option. While Dr. Singleton and I know from both personal and clinical experience that acupuncture works, it pleases me that the NIH now formally recognizes the merits of this treatment.

▲▲▲▲▲▲▲▲▲▲▲▲▲▲▲▲▲▲▲▲▲▲▲▲▲▲▲▲▲▲

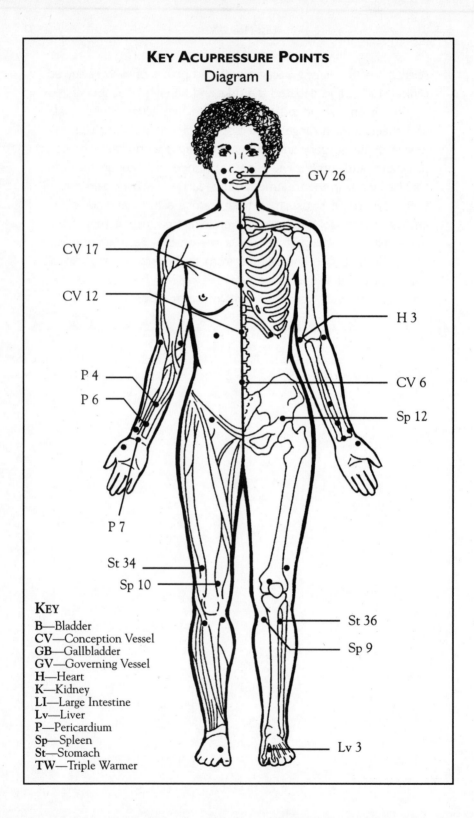

KEY ACUPRESSURE POINTS
Diagram I

GV 26

CV 17

CV 12

H 3

P 4

CV 6

P 6

Sp 12

P 7

St 34

Sp 10

St 36

Sp 9

Lv 3

KEY
B—Bladder
CV—Conception Vessel
GB—Gallbladder
GV—Governing Vessel
H—Heart
K—Kidney
LI—Large Intestine
Lv—Liver
P—Pericardium
Sp—Spleen
St—Stomach
TW—Triple Warmer

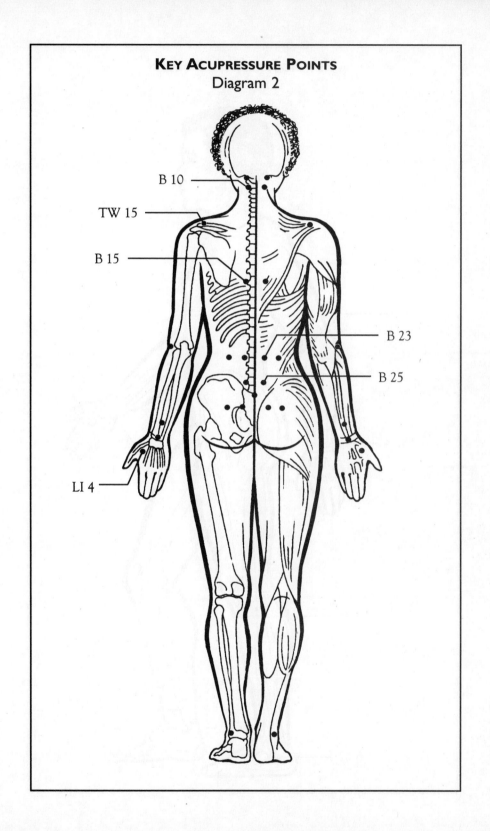

KEY ACUPRESSURE POINTS
Diagram 2

B 10

TW 15

B 15

B 23

B 25

LI 4

KEY ACUPRESSURE POINTS
Diagram 3

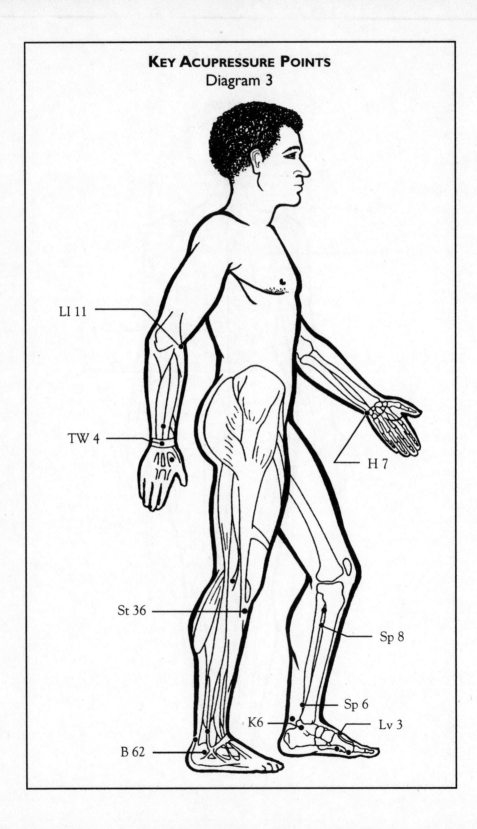

LI 11

TW 4

H 7

St 36

Sp 8

Sp 6

K6

Lv 3

B 62

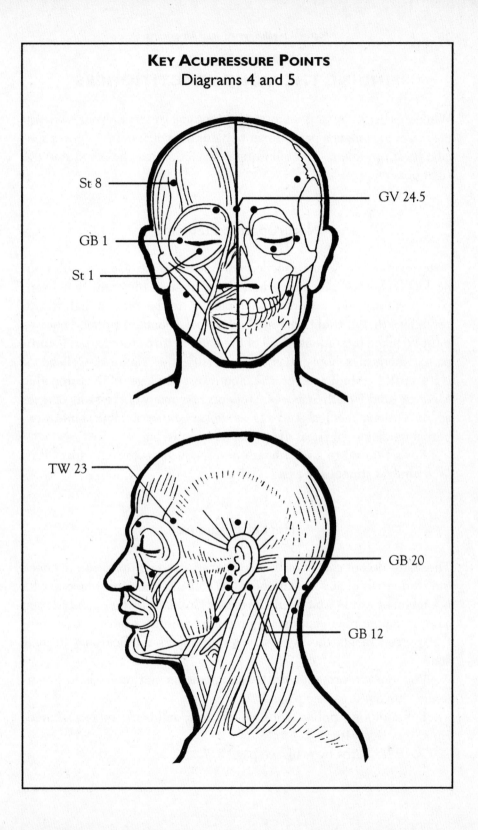

KEY ACUPRESSURE POINTS
Diagrams 4 and 5

St 8

GV 24.5

GB 1

St 1

TW 23

GB 20

GB 12

FINDING THE RIGHT PRACTITIONERS

While this book contains many suggestions you can try on your own, you may want to contact a practitioner of natural medicine if you have a specific health problem. The following information may help you find the right person:

Naturopathic Medicine

Naturopathic physicians practice natural medicine using a variety of healing techniques, including herbalism, homeopathy, nutritional supplementation, and acupressure. Training to become a naturopath resembles that in traditional medical school. Standard premed courses must be taken by students at all of the nation's three recognized naturopathic medical schools, Bastyr University, the National College of Naturopathic Medicine, or the Southwest College of Naturopathic Medicine and Health Sciences. Students take many of the same courses as conventional medical students, as well as courses in clinical nutrition, herbal medicine, physical medicine, and counseling.

For a referral to a naturopath or a medical doctor who specializes in natural treatments, see page 315.

Herbal Medicine

The states do not certify or license herbalists, so it's up to you to check the credentials of any practitioners you consult. Look for someone who is a member of the American Herbalists Guild, or if you're considering a naturopathic physician or acupuncturist who uses herbs, make sure that person meets the necessary requirements for licensing in your state.

For more information on herbal medicine and referrals to practitioners in your area, see page 315.

For additional publications, newsletters, and books on herbal medicine, see page 316.

To order herbs by mail, see page 317.

Diet and Nutrition

If you have special nutritional needs or want to design a regimen of nutrition supplements to help manage your specific health needs, you may want to consult a nutrition counselor. For information on finding a qualified nutritionist, see page 318.

For publications on nutrition (some for a fee), see page 319.

Homeopathy

Homeopathy is considered the practice of medicine and it can be performed legally only by medical professionals. The requirements for licensure vary from state to state. While medical doctors (M.D.s) and osteopaths (D.O.s) can practice homeopathy in all states, many other medical professionals—such as naturopaths (N.D.s) and chiropractors (D.C.s)—may be qualified to practice homeopathy, provided they meet the necessary licensing requirements. There are many other trained homeopaths who do not fall into these categories; some may do a good job and others may not. Ask about a practitioner's training and experience before making an appointment.

For an information packet on homeopathy and a directory of practitioners, see page 320.

You may also want to buy homeopathic remedies for home treatment of many common ailments. For manufacturers who supply homeopathic remedies by mail, see page 320.

Acupuncture and Acupressure

While you can practice acupressure as a self-help technique, you may want to consult a professional if you have additional questions or if you would like to try acupuncture for a more powerful healing effect.

Nationwide, approximately three thousand medical doctors and osteopaths have studied acupuncture and use it as one of the tools in their medical practice. An additional seven thousand naturopaths and acupuncturists use the techniques. Medicaid and a number of private insurance companies cover acupuncture in some circumstances; check with your insurance company before consulting a professional to find out whether the treatment will be covered. Treatment usually costs $40 to $100 for the initial visit and $30 to $70 for follow-up sessions; physician acupuncturists may cost more.

Acupuncture and acupressure professionals must meet state licensing or certification requirements in twenty-nine states and the District of Columbia. All states allow medical doctors to practice acupuncture, but only fourteen require physicians to have formal training in it.

If you want to use a physician acupuncturist or acupressurist, look for someone who is a member of the American Academy of Medical Acupuncture. To become a member, a physician must complete at least two hundred hours of acupuncture training and have two years of clinical experience. Approximately three thousand doctors practice acupuncture in the United States today, but only about 1000 of them are AAMA members. The AAMA also has a certification examination; practitioners are required to practice for two years before they are eligible to take the exam.

For more information or a referral, see page 323.

If you're interested in seeing a nonphysician acupuncturist or acupressurist, make sure they have been certified by the National Commission for the Certification of Acupuncturists. (A certified member can use the title Diplomate of Acupuncture, indicated by the initials Dipl.Ac. after his or her name.) To become certified, an acupuncturist must pass both a written and practical exam; to be eligible to take the exams, he or she must be licensed, must have at least three years of training, or must have worked as an apprentice acupuncturist for at least four years. For more information or to confirm certification of a particular acupuncturist or acupressurist, see page 323.

For additional information on acupuncture and acupressure, as well as for a free referral to practitioners in your area, see page 323.

3

▼

Mind, Body, Spirit, Soul

Redefining What It Means to Be Healthy

If a picture paints a thousand words, then firsthand experience must be worth about a million words. Rather than simply explaining to you the interconnectedness of the mind and body, we would like to show you. Before reading on, please track down a friend or partner and perform this experiment. It will take only about five minutes.

▼▼▼▼▼▼▼▼▼▼▼▼▼▼▼▼▼▼▼▼▼▼▼▼

EMOTIONS AND HEALTH

Stand facing your partner with one arm held straight out to your side at a ninety-degree angle. Your partner should place his or her hand on top of your extended wrist and push down on your arm as you resist with all your might. In essence, your partner is assessing the strength of your deltoid muscle.

Now we would like you to pause and think of a negative experience, perhaps something that happened in the past week that either hurt you or made you very angry. Think about this experience for sixty to ninety seconds, then extend your arm and repeat the deltoid strength test.

41

Were your muscles stronger or weaker? Why do you think your body responded as it did?

Now repeat the exercise, only this time think of an experience that made you feel happy, proud, loved. What happened this time?

▲▲▲▲▲▲▲▲▲▲▲▲▲▲▲▲▲▲▲▲▲▲▲▲▲▲▲▲▲

Most people believe that they will become stronger or more powerful when they experience anger. Anger is seen as empowering in our society, but the opposite is true. Most people who perform this little experiment find that their arm is much weaker when they are caught up in anger or a negative thought; it is more difficult to hold up your arm because your energy is drained. It is often difficult to appreciate how much energy our anger and negative emotions take from us until we see the point demonstrated to us.

Over time, chronic anger can weaken our immune system and lead to illness. The problem is not with the expression of anger; the problem is the injury to the body that comes if we are not willing to resolve or release the anger so we can reclaim the energy that is below the anger. (For a longer discussion on anger, see page 60.)

THE MIND-BODY LINK

Western culture tries to separate the body and the mind, but as both medical doctors and practitioners of "alternative" medicine, we respect, acknowledge, and celebrate the interconnectedness of the mind and body. Though many people think of Eastern techniques when they consider mind-body healing, African shamans and medicine men traditionally used dance and ritual to bring forth the spirit and use its powerful force in healing. Our ancestors believed that all organs in the human body are related to one another; just as all organs evolved from a single fertilized egg, so the organs have maintained their connection to the whole body. This holistic approach to health is part of the African philosophy of healing.

We have seen evidence of the mind-body link time and again in our medical practices. One of the most common mind-body illnesses involves migraine headache. Consider the twenty-eight-year-old African American woman who came to the office complaining of severe migraines. She took multiple medications for the condition, but they were not very effective at controlling her pain. After speaking with her, we noted that the headaches followed a clear pattern: She would invariably experience a migraine when things were not going well in her relationship with her husband.

During one visit, we prayed together and the woman remembered being very young and witnessing a severe beating her mother had received at her father's hand. She began working on forgiving her father, and her migraines became less frequent. She soon went off all the medication, and she now has only occasional migraines.

This woman used her mind to heal her body, but the mind can also be used to undermine the healing process. Often when African Americans, especially those in the inner city, are diagnosed with a chronic or potentially fatal disease, they give up and say "it's just my time" to die. They resign themselves to the worst, and all too often their expectations are fulfilled.

The importance of attitude has even been quantified in the laboratory. A 1990 study done at the University of Pittsburgh School of Medicine found that patients with breast cancer who felt emotionally supported had vigorous natural killer cells (white blood cells that help destroy tumor cells) compared to their unsupported counterparts. The same year, researchers at the UCLA/Neuropsychiatric Institute found that people with malignant melanoma who participated in counseling sessions for six weeks had lower levels of psychological distress, better coping skills, and more active natural killer cells than people who did not receive counseling. Five years later, the members of the support group had significantly higher survival rates compared to people who did not join in the support groups. Another study done at the University of Pittsburgh, Carnegie Mellon University, and the University of Georgia found that among cancer patients under age sixty, a pessimistic outlook has a direct and detrimental effect on how long a patient survives.

While the mind-body connection is nothing new, Western scientists "discovered" it about twenty-five years ago. Back in 1974, psychologist Robert Ader, M.D., Ph.D., performed a simple experiment designed to teach rats to avoid drinking sweetened water. What his experiment actually established was the link between the mind and body. As part of the experiment, Ader put sweet, saccharin-flavored water in the rats' cages, and each time they drank from it he gave them a drug that made them feel nauseous. Later in the experiment, the rats were given the sweetened water without the upsetting drug; those rats that drank the water acted as though they had received the drug, and many became sick and died.

Surprised by the results of his experiment, Ader further investigated the drug he was using and discovered that it suppressed the immune system in addition to causing nausea. Ultimately he concluded that the rats had learned to voluntarily suppress their immune systems in response to the sugar water because they had established a mental link between sweet water and immune suppression. This landmark study was the first to demonstrate in a laboratory the powerful link between the mind and body.

Since then, a new interdisciplinary field of medicine called psychoneuroimmunology (PNI) has emerged. This complex field examines how psychological and behavioral issues influence the course of diseases of the immune system. It is the Western medical establishment's way of exploring the inextricable connections between the mind and body and health and illness.

PNI researchers have learned a lot about the mind-body link, though there is much that remains a mystery. Scientists have demonstrated that the nervous system and the immune system communicate using a complex chemical network of neurotransmitters, hormones, and neuropeptides. To be technical, we know that when the body is stressed, the hypothalamus in the brain produces a corticotropin-releasing factor, which in turn triggers the secretion of adrenocorticotropic hormones. These hormones cause the adrenal system to release corticosteroid hormones, which suppress the immune system and make the body more susceptible to illness. In other words, stress contributes to immune suppression and illness.

Of course, we need to avoid the temptation to make something very complex into something very simple. When it comes to health, almost every problem is multifaceted. In addition to the stress and psychological issues, our bodies also respond to a number of other factors that affect our health, such as genetics, age, sex, personality, environment, bacteria, viruses, carcinogens, medical care, and socioeconomic factors, to name just a few. Our behavior also affects our immune system; smoking ciga-rettes, drinking alcohol, getting enough rest, eating or not eating right—these factors also contribute to the strength of our immune system.

We must learn to appreciate the influence of the mind on the body without trying to turn it into a monolithic theory, one that assumes the mind alone can control overall health. Rather than replacing one restricting approach to healing with another, we must be open to accepting a holistic view of the body, which sees the mind as one of many factors that can influence overall health.

▼▼▼▼▼▼▼▼▼▼▼▼▼▼▼▼▼▼▼▼▼▼▼▼▼▼

OUR HISTORY OF HEALING

The ancient Egyptians did not separate the mind and the body. Instead, they would describe organs of the body as having mental or spiritual qualities, though they also understood that there was a unity between the body, mind, emotions, and spirit. Many people living in the Western world do not explicitly acknowledge this mind-body connection, though most of us do seem to intuitively know it. Even today we say things like "He didn't have his heart in it" or "I can feel it in my bones."

▲▲▲▲▲▲▲▲▲▲▲▲▲▲▲▲▲▲▲▲▲▲▲▲▲▲

THE ROLE OF STRESS

Of the thousands of patients we have admitted to the hospital over the years because of medical illness, all have one thing in common: When asked if anything unusual happened just before they got sick, they all complained that they were under a lot of stress. Stress can make us sick.

Stress is part of being alive; it cannot be avoided. If you lived on a desert island, you would have stress; if you were a millionaire, you would have stress; if you had a secure job with fabulous benefits, you would have stress. No matter what you do, stress can always find you.

The challenges of living aren't stressful in themselves; it's how you react to those events that causes stress. Our attitudes, expectations, past experiences, perceptions, and personality have a lot to do with how we handle stress—and how our bodies respond to it. People with poor coping skills experience more harmful immune-system changes in response to stress than those who learn to manage their emotions. In fact, people who can handle stress or perceive it as a positive challenge can actually grow from stress.

Those people who cope well with stress have what psychologist Suzanne Kobasa of the City University of New York calls "hardiness." While at the University of Chicago, Kobasa studied businessmen and the ways they managed corporate stress. She found that those who stayed healthiest saw their work as a challenge (rather than a threat) and felt in control of the decisions they made.

Other researchers have found a high rate of heart disease risk factors associated with high-pressure, low-control jobs. For example, one study found that bus drivers, secretaries, and air traffic controllers (all jobs with lots of pressure and little control) were among the professionals most likely to have high blood pressure and an enlargement of the left ventricular area of the heart.

Of course, not all stress is bad. Without stress, there would be little positive change. Stress can be caused by the environment (air and noise pollution, overcrowding, weather) as well as by both distressing or even pleasurable experiences. In fact, positive experiences can be just as physically stressful as negative ones.

When the body perceives stress, it kicks into the so-called fight or flight response, which involves a number of biochemical changes that happen in preparation for dealing with danger. In evolutionary terms, this high-intensity state makes sense because quick bursts of energy were required to fight off predators or flee a dangerous situation. Of course, in our daily lives we face fewer of these life-or-death threats, but the modern world remains full of stressors—financial worries, subways, children, health concerns, deadline pressures, relationship problems. When confronted with these contemporary stressors, our bodies respond in much the same way as those of our prehistoric ancestors once did.

Much of the stress we experience in our daily lives cannot be managed by either fighting or fleeing; when your boss yells at you about a missed deadline you can neither assault him nor turn and run away. Instead, you do all you can to internalize your emotions and suppress your anger, fear, self-blame, or whatever else you might be feeling in order to keep your job. Despite your external control, internally your body has entered a state of high-stress preparedness.

In the body, any stressor—either real or imagined—triggers an alarm in the hypothalamus in the midbrain. The hypothalamus then shifts into overdrive, warning the body that it must prepare for an emergency. As a result, your heart races, your breathing speeds up, your muscles tense, your metabolism kicks into high gear, and your blood pressure soars. Your blood concentrates in your muscles, leaving your hands and feet cold and your muscles ready for action. Your senses become more acute: Your hearing becomes sharper and your pupils dilate. You're ready to fight or flee.

As part of the intricate system of stress response, your body also releases adrenaline, epinephrine, cortisol, and other chemicals that inhibit the immune system and interfere with digestion, reproduction, growth, and tissue repair. While not harmful in short bursts, these stress responses can cause serious health problems if the stress continues for long periods of time. For example, someone working in a high-stress job, going through a difficult divorce, or recovering from abuse as a child might experience the physiological effects of stress for a prolonged period.

Over the long haul, these stress responses can contribute to the development of disease. Chronic stress can elevate blood pressure, contributing to hypertension; it can cause muscle tension, resulting in headaches and digestive disorders; it can suppress the immune system, leaving an individual prone to colds, flus, and a range of serious diseases. Stress can cause a number of specific illnesses, such as depression, irritable bowel syndrome, and other gastrointestinal disorders. A study done by the U.S. Department of Health and Human Services Epidemiology Center in Atlanta, Georgia, found that during periods of national economic instability or recession, there was a marked increase in the number of people who experienced peptic ulcers, heart attacks, impotence, and weight loss, to name a few.

Because of the harmful effects of long-term, internalized stress, it is essential for your health that you find ways to express your emotions and to release the physical effects of stress. Fortunately, a systematic approach to stress management and natural healing can help control and overcome these health problems. Chapter 4, "Attitude Is Everything," page 59, provides techniques to help you express your emotions and release stress.

Stress-reduction techniques helped a fifty-two-year-old African American woman who experienced recurrent abdominal pain episodes. At times this woman's pain was so great that she required hospitalization. After performing a battery of tests (all of which showed no physical problem), we taught her the classic stress-reduction techniques, in addition to prescribing acupuncture and nutritional supplements. When she came to us she admitted that she had been quite worried about the granddaughter she was raising. Her life still presents challenges, of course, but she uses her new skills to manage the physical symptoms of stress. She is doing well and rarely experiences stomach pains.

STRIVE TO HEAL, NOT TO CURE

One truth that we try to help our patients understand is that it is possible to be *healed* without being *cured*. To be cured means that the illness or physical problem that has plagued you has disappeared; to be healed means that the way you hold the illness in your consciousness has shifted.

For example, if you happen to have sickle-cell disease, you can be healed, though there may be nothing you can do to alter your body's genetic makeup. In this case, to be healed you must move to a place where on an emotional, mental, and spiritual level you are released of negative feelings about what having sickle-cell disease means to you. Perhaps in your mind this condition makes you feel uncomfortable about your ancestry and your past; healing can take place when you learn to let go of those negative feelings. You are healed when you evolve into a whole and beautiful being who is in touch with your own loving; at that point, the sickle-cell disease loses its power to get in the way of loving yourself.

In effect, having sickle-cell disease may become the vehicle or the catalyst that allows you to get in touch with who you really are. The sickle-cell disease can lose its previous meaning and become the respected and positive force in your life that helped you transform your image of yourself for the better. In this way, a person can be healed, even if an illness cannot be cured.

This concept was difficult for one patient—a divorced young mother with several children—to understand. The woman had custody of her children, but her ex-husband had visitation rights. Each time the couple saw each other, they fought. The woman was so filled with hatred and anger toward her former spouse that she would spend ten to twenty hours per week wrangling over court dates and fighting over unpaid child support.

What happened, of course, was that the woman paid the price for her anger. She had migraine headaches almost daily; she couldn't gain weight; she was severely depressed; she always arrived at the office weeping and an emotional wreck. She never resolved her feelings for her ex-husband and sought negative attention from him (it was, after all, better than being forgotten, according to her unconscious logic).

As we started to work with her feelings about her ex-husband, the woman began to see that all of the physical symptoms that she was having were directly related to the stress and energy drain that she was creating for herself. She thought that she needed her ex-husband to make her whole by either repairing the broken relationship or by validating her emotions, but she eventually realized that she could set herself free, like Dorothy in the Wizard of Oz. Her ex-husband was no longer the problem (he was out of her life); the problem had become the woman's desire to prove to her ex-husband that he had wronged her. Once she saw that it was her unresolved anger that was stopping her from moving forward, she got in touch with the hurt and feelings of abandonment, and no longer needed to feel trapped by these negative emotions. As the anger disappeared, so did her physical symptoms.

HEALING AND BELONGING

A growing body of evidence suggests that positive social support is necessary for a person's health. The sense of belonging and affiliation appears to be a basic human need. There is now abundant evidence to show that social support may be one of the critical elements distinguishing those who remain healthy from those who do not.

Both the positive and the negative influences of social support have been documented. Positive and supportive associations, such as community support and close friends or family, have been linked to better overall heath, lower incidence of cancer and heart disease, and reduced hospital stays. We all need a sense of being connected.

The lack of social stability and social connectedness (sometimes called "social marginality") have been linked to a variety of behavioral, physical, and psychological illnesses, including arthritis, tuberculosis, hypertension, schizophrenia, depression, coronary disease, and general mortality rates.

Theories about social support in humans have been supported by animal research. When subjected to stressful situations, animals with familiar "cage mates" have been found to be more able to cope with hypertension, cancer, negative stressors, and maternal separation. This animal research suggests that networks of social support may have evolved to sustain health. We used to live in tribes or communities in which we all supported one another, which helped reduce stress. As people have become more isolated from their extended families and their communities, stress and disease have increased.

▼▼▼▼▼▼▼▼▼▼▼▼▼▼▼▼▼▼▼▼▼▼▼▼▼

CONSIDER THE EVIDENCE

A number of fascinating studies have been conducted around the world supporting the mind-body connection. Following are just a few:

- People with multiple personality disorder exhibit different allergic reactions, sexual preferences, patterns of addiction, diabetic reactions, and visual acuity when different personalities are present. Electroencephalographic recordings are as statistically different among personalities as they are among different individuals.

- According to a study reported in the *Archives of Internal Medicine,* researchers at the University of Arkansas College of Medicine worked with a thirty-nine-year-old woman who was an experienced meditator. Using meditation and visualization, she was able to voluntarily delay her sensitivity to a skin test using a virus that causes the skin to blister. Other studies have found that experienced meditators can voluntarily control their pain, bleeding, and infection following self-inflicted puncture wounds.

- Stress can cause birth defects. A 1995 study conducted at the University of Chile, Santiago, looked at the health impact of a large earthquake (9 on the Richter scale) that took place on March 2, 1985, in Santiago, Chile. The researchers reviewed the characteristics of more than 22,000 births registered at three public hospitals later that year. They found a significant increase in the rate of facial clefts—2.01 per 1,000 births in contrast to 1.6 per 1,000 births in previous years. The increase was greatest (3.8 per 1,000 births) in those babies born in September (these mothers were in their first trimester at the time of the stressful earthquake). The researchers suspect that the increase in clefting could be an unwanted side effect of the stress the mothers experienced during the earthquake.

- A 1996 study conducted by Duke University Medical Center researchers found that patients with a history of coronary artery disease who are mentally stressed are almost three times more likely to suffer a serious cardiac event than those who aren't. More than 27 percent of those patients who became stressed during the tests (which included tasks such as giving a short speech, reading aloud, and performing serial additions) experienced a significant cardiac event compared to only 12 percent of those who stayed calm under pressure.

- Several studies have looked at the impact of academic examinations and changes in immune functioning. One study found a decrease in the secretion of the immune-enhancing immunoglobulin-A during periods of academic stress in first-year dental students compared to periods of little academic stress. Other studies found similar results when looking at medical students on the first day of final exams. During the exam period, these students produce less interferon and natural killer cells, indicating a weakened immune system.

- Studies on bereavement suggest that the stress of losing a loved one may inhibit the formation of immune-enhancing lymphocytes. One study reported a significant drop in lymphocytes eight weeks after the loss of a spouse.

- A study conducted at Boston University found that university students who were shown a film about Mother Teresa's work taking care of the sick and poor in Calcutta, India, experienced a boost in their immune systems. This immune system enhancement occurred whether or not the students approved of her work.

▲▲▲▲▲▲▲▲▲▲▲▲▲▲▲▲▲▲▲▲▲▲▲▲▲▲▲▲▲▲▲▲

LETTING GO OF STRESS

Fortunately, the stress response can be easily reversed. Your body begins to relax as soon as your brain receives the signal that the danger has passed and it's safe to calm down. About three minutes after the brain cancels the emergency signals to the central nervous system, the panic messages cease and relaxation begins. Your heart rate and breathing gradually slow down, and your other systems return to their normal levels.

You can actually teach yourself how to promote the relaxation response by using the techniques discussed in Chapter 4, "Attitude Is Everything: Living with Stress, Prejudice, and Negative Emotions," page 59. These simple exercises will allow you to use your mind to soothe and heal your body.

▼▼▼▼▼▼▼▼▼▼▼▼▼▼▼▼▼▼▼▼▼▼▼▼▼▼

IT'S ALL IN YOUR HEAD

The mind can be helpful in healing—but it also can contribute to the development of psychological or psychosomatic illness. In such cases, the person confronts a stressful situation that cannot be easily resolved. At some point, the situation becomes overwhelming and the person attempts to resolve the problem the only way considered possible—the unconscious mind makes the person sick. For example, he might develop a migraine headache so severe that it puts him in bed; he has become incapacitated and can no longer perform the responsibilities that have caused so much stress. The illness has allowed the person to escape an untenable situation he could not resolve by other means.

If the approach is effective—and it often is—the same pattern of illness resurfaces when the stress reappears. This pattern is a learned response that often begins in childhood. Fortunately, just as it has been learned, it can be unlearned.

People with psychosomatic illness aren't faking; they really do have the symptoms they report. However, the illness involves a complex interaction of the mind and body, and it will require a more holistic approach to healing. Only by understanding the root cause of the problem can the afflicted person become healed. While Western medicine may help to alleviate some of the symptoms (and it may not), the practice of stress-reduction techniques can be much more helpful in the prevention of psychosomatic disease in the first place. And, of course, there are times when the help of a qualified therapist can focus the healing process and speed your recovery.

▲▲▲▲▲▲▲▲▲▲▲▲▲▲▲▲▲▲▲▲▲▲▲▲▲▲

▼▼▼▼▼▼▼▼▼▼▼▼▼▼▼▼▼▼▼▼▼

HOW STRESSED ARE YOU?

Stress can make you sick. Studies have found a strong correlation between the intensity and stress of life changes and the onset of severe illness. Years ago several researchers devised the Social Readjustment Rating Scale, a chart that assigns numerical values to common stressful events. They include both disappointments (distress)—such as job loss, death of a close friend, injury, and so on—and joyful events (eustress)—such as marriage, pregnancy, new job, and so on. Both types of experience cause stress and require adjustment.

To use the chart, circle the events that have occurred in your life in the past year and add up the numerical values assigned to these events. Based on their study, the researchers determined that if you received a score of 150, your chances of developing an illness would be roughly 50-50. If you were to score over 300 points within a year, your chances of experiencing some kind of health change go up to almost 90 percent. As the score increases, the probability that the health change would be a serious illness increases also.

SOCIAL READJUSTMENT RATING SCALE

Event	Value
Death of spouse	100
Divorce	73
Marital separation	65
Jail term	63
Death of a close family member	63
Personal injury or illness	53
Marriage	50

Fired from work	47
Marital reconciliation	45
Retirement	45
Change in family member's health	44
Pregnancy	40
Sex difficulties	39
Addition to family	39
Business readjustment	39
Change in financial status	38
Death of a close friend	37
Change to different line of work	36
Change in number of marital arguments	35
Mortgage or loan over $10,000	31
Foreclosure of mortgage or loan	30
Change in work responsibilities	29
Son or daughter leaving home	29
Trouble with in-laws	29
Outstanding personal achievement	28
Spouse begins or stops work	26
Starting or finishing school	26
Change in living conditions	25
Revision of personal habits	24
Trouble with boss	23
Change in work hours, conditions	20
Change in residence	20
Change in schools	20
Change in recreation habits	19
Change in church activities	19
Change in social activities	18
Mortgages or loan under $10,000	17
Change in sleeping habits	16
Change in number of family gatherings	15
Change in eating habits	15
Vacation	13
Christmas season	12
Minor violation of the law	11

▼▼▼▼▼▼▼▼▼▼▼▼▼▼▼▼▼▼

PART 2

Nurturing Ourselves

▲▲▲▲▲▲▲▲▲▲▲▲▲▲▲▲▲▲

4
▼

Attitude Is Everything

Living with Stress, Prejudice, and Negative Emotions

Being black in America is stressful, no matter what your profession, age, or economic status. We see evidence of the health hazards of stress in our patients time and again: Racial prejudice—both overt and covert—whittles away self-esteem and contributes to stress-related illness. In addition, violence both inside and outside the home leaves many African Americans with the perception that there is no safe refuge from stress. (For more information on the physical effects of stress on the body, see Chapter 3, "Mind, Body, Spirit, Soul," page 41.)

So why is it that some African Americans can be exposed to these stresses and maintain an inner calm and serenity, while others become ill and grow angry and perpetuate or magnify the violence? Your disposition has something to do with how you respond to stress, but you can learn to handle stress and avoid its negative impact on your body and your life by practicing some specific and simple stress-reduction techniques. We have had a lot of success teaching our patients how to defuse stress by using the practices described in this chapter.

UNDERSTANDING ANGER

As African Americans, we all encounter prejudice and racism, but as individuals we have a personal choice about how we react to these experiences. If you receive anger or hostility from someone else, you can choose to let the anger pass through you, or you can hold on to it and make it your own. Unfortunately, many people respond to anger with anger.

In the spectrum of human emotion, anger is probably the least understood. Anger is neither a sign of weakness nor a measure of strength; it is, however, a powerful form of energy. Anger is hot, like the steam inside a pot, and it wants to expand, to push the lid off the pot and escape. We all feel anger to varying degrees; our personal challenge is to find constructive ways of dealing with this expansive and moving form of emotional energy.

Problems with anger arise when anger leads to destructive practices, such as emotional, mental, or physical abuse. Many people make quick decisions or say things they later regret, only to feel ashamed or defensive after the episode has passed. If your expression of anger is harmful to you or others, you need to learn new ways of expressing this powerful emotion.

Here are four common ways people deal with anger:

- **Explosion.** This expression of anger is emotion in motion; it is a blowout that can be very harmful, especially if it is directed at another person. Some people explode and then the anger passes; others explode and smolder. Explosions can injure the person feeling the anger, as well at those who get in the way. If you tend to explode with anger, reflect on how these episodes make you feel about yourself. When the moment passes, do you say to yourself, "I should not have done that"? If you do, then the anger has passed but a judgment about yourself remains. You need to find healthier ways to express your anger.

- **Repression.** Unexpressed anger is repressed anger. Some people can internalize their anger so well that people around them do not know that they are upset, and in some cases people fool themselves into believing that they are not angry. Anger can be a frightening emotion for people uncomfortable with its intensity. The problem with repressed anger is that the anger is turned back inside the person who feels angry. Many African Americans don't vent their anger very well. Instead, their negative feelings go inward and lead to health problems such as hypertension, stroke, depression, neck pain, addiction, and heart disease, to name just a few. Of course, not everyone who experiences these illnesses has a problem with repressed anger, but if you have recurrent health problems, you should ask yourself if you are angry about something. Assess your feelings and decide if you are not acknowledging your anger (or other emotions). While many people think this process takes years of psychotherapy or counseling, it all comes down to a single moment of conscious choice: I choose to heal, I choose to tell myself the absolute truth about how I am feeling. Look for feelings of fear and jealousy; many childhood emotions are at the root of our adult anger.

- **Suppression.** Suppression is like repression, except that the person who is suppressing his or her anger knows what they are feeling and chooses to withhold the emotions. Some people suppress their anger by avoiding the person causing it; others simply refuse to speak their mind. This approach to managing anger creates a separation between you and the person you are angry with. If you feel distant from someone you care about, ask yourself if you are suppressing your emotions. Focus on what you are feeling and begin to think about ways you can share your true feelings.

- **Depression.** While many cases of depression can involve biochemical imbalances in the brain, in some cases depression can also be an expression of repressed rage. It takes a tremendous amount of energy to bottle up this powerful emotion, and doing so can cause some people to withdraw from the world and lose interest in others and activities. By learning to release this anger in a safe and positive way, some people will find relief from their depression.

Do you see yourself in any of these examples? If you recognize that you have a problem with anger, first we want to commend you for your willingness to work on the problem. Next it is important to understand what makes us angry. In most cases, anger comes from how we feel about ourselves; we become angry when there is a gap between what we feel we should be and what we believe that we are. If you run the hundred-yard dash and come in first place, you probably won't be angry. But if you disappoint yourself or fail to live up to your vision of what you want to be, then you may feel angry. If someone says something hurtful to you or cuts you off in traffic, you may become angry because this experience does not match your vision of how you wish to be treated.

Some outbreaks of anger disintegrate as soon as the moment passes, but others we hold on to for months, years—even a lifetime. Many of the patients who have trouble with anger cannot let go of a situation that may have happened long ago. That's because beneath the anger is pain—the pain of not living up to our goals, the pain of rejection, the pain of loneliness. We must dig behind the anger to discover the source of the pain that keeps the anger alive.

Finally, beneath the hurt is another emotion: love—love of self, love of another, love of the universe. There is no simple formula for reaching the love: You have to choose it and it will come to you. Once you reach the point of emotional truth with yourself, the love can be uncovered.

Many of our patients ask, "How can anger be so closely related to love?" We respond, "How is an atom related to a bomb?" The potential emotional energy is enormous; the issue involves how that energy is harnessed and directed. Once you look beneath the anger to the hurt and then beneath the hurt to the love, you can reach a place where there is peace and tranquillity. If you could release the enormous weight of your anger, just imagine how much lighter you would feel. Only by working through the anger can you experience healing and reach a place of truly knowing and loving yourself.

WORKING THROUGH YOUR ANGER AND NEGATIVE EMOTIONS

The question, of course, is what can you do to let go of the anger and negative emotions? To release yourself from anger, you need to acknowledge it and express it in a way that allows you to be heard (without hurting you or anyone else in the process). Part of the healing process involves finding constructive ways to deal with anger and negative emotions. To do this, you need to learn certain skills.

The first thing you need to do is tell yourself the truth. This may sound simple but it is sometimes one of the most difficult things we can do. It can be helpful to start with a simple statement like "I am angry because of . . ." Be gentle with yourself; some of the intense emotions you feel may make you uncomfortable.

The next thing to do is to not try to dismiss your anger and pain. All too often when people tell themselves the truth about their feelings, they immediately try to tell themselves that they have moved beyond the pain—"I'm over it already." It would be nice if working through pain were so quick and tidy; unfortunately, in most cases it isn't that simple. You will know that the issue has not been resolved if you still feel bad about yourself over the issue. If you still experience some judgment about yourself, there is more work to be done.

Fortunately, there are specific things you can do to deal constructively with anger. Here are a few suggestions:

- **Free-form writing.** Pick up a piece of paper and a pen and start writing down what you feel. The words you write don't need to make sense; you don't need to worry about grammar, spelling, or editing. You don't even need to reread what you write. All you need is paper and a pen and the freedom to allow yourself to express all of your feelings openly. Write until you feel that the anger has dissolved and you can feel an emotional shift inside you. It may take one page, or it may take many. Just keep going; you deserve all the time this may take.

  A literary purge can free you up emotionally. As you honestly vent your feelings and give your anger "a voice," the anger will pass and the underlying hurt and sadness will surface. And once you see and understand where the pain is really coming from, you can take steps to apply loving and healing to that part of yourself that may feel broken or damaged. We often have a tendency to disallow or ignore those parts of ourselves that make us feel weak, vulnerable, or in pain. However, once the process of healing has begun, we can slowly get in touch with the feelings that we have disowned (and perhaps feared), allowing us to once again feel whole.

When you have finished this exercise, ball up the paper and burn it or tear it into tiny pieces. The words you write are not meant to be shared; they are meant to give voice to your feelings.

- **Exercise.** Physical exercise is constructive expression of the moving energy of anger and negative emotions. When you feel anger, move your body: Dance, run, pull weeds, do karate, hit a baseball, whack a pillow. (Sex is not included on this list because it involves channeling your anger through someone else.) As long as the physical motion of your anger isn't harmful to you, to others, or to the things around you, use your body to express yourself.

- **Role play.** It can be very cathartic to have an imaginary conversation. Imagine that the person you are angry with is sitting in a chair, then yell and scream at the empty chair. (Remember, your goal is not to have others experience your wrath but to move through your anger so the other person does not need to be involved.)

    Tell the imaginary person how you feel; tell them how their actions or abuse hurt you. This approach can be used to confront someone who has died, someone who is not available to you because they are in a position of authority, or someone who is unavailable for any of a number of other reasons.

    This technique can be very powerful. Be careful; it can stir up a lot of emotional energy. It is a particularly energetic exercise because your energy is directed at the person who has offended or hurt you. If you feel you have a great deal of unexpressed anger, it may be more effective and nurturing for you to do this work with a therapist or a professional "anger workshop" facilitator.

- **Join a support group.** Talk about your feelings in a safe network or group where you can express yourself freely, knowing that anything you say will be honored, respected, and kept confidential.

- **Keep a journal.** Record your experiences and feelings in a diary or journal. With free-form writing, the words you write are not important; the process of writing is what frees you. (Some people even burn or throw away their writings when they have finished.) On the other hand, journaling is intended to be read and referred to as part of the healing process. Each day, you record your feelings and experiences, and every week or so you look back over your writings and reflect on what has happened, remaining open to recognizing patterns and receiving insights about yourself.

- **Tell your side of the story.** If you have been hurt by someone, write a letter that you will never send (if the person will not see the letter, you will feel freer to be honest). Explain your position and point out all of your good qualities that the person overlooked. It can be a relief to defend yourself, even if you aren't able to express yourself directly to the person who hurt you. When you're doing this exercise, it is important to state the specific behavior that bothered you, followed by how you felt when it happened. For example, "When you were an hour late and didn't call, I felt afraid."

- **Rewrite history.** Visualize the negative encounter or the experience that has hurt you and this time reframe the whole event as if it happened a different way. This exercise takes advantage of the fact that the human brain has a hard time distinguishing between what really happened and your revision of history.

After you allow your anger to come to the surface and to be expressed, the next thing to do is to determine whether you are holding any negative judgments against yourself. So often when we receive negative emotions, we internalize them with self-judgment. If you were raped, you might feel damaged or dirty; if you were criticized, you might feel ugly or stupid.

Once you understand the ways you judge yourself, you can move into the stage of self-forgiveness. The process of forgiveness is simple (but may take some practice):

- Recognize the judgments you hold about yourself.

- List them: I feel dirty; I feel damaged; I feel ugly; I feel stupid.

- Say (aloud) that you forgive yourself for those feelings. "I forgive myself for judging myself as dirty." "I forgive myself for judging myself as damaged."

Sometimes it can be helpful to look at a picture of yourself at the age you were at the time you made this judgment about yourself; stare at the picture as you offer your statement of self-forgiveness aloud.

You may also find it helpful to give yourself affirmations (to recite statements to build your self-confidence). Affirmations are short, positive statements you tell yourself that help you see yourself in a positive way. They should be specific, based in the present (not the future), and they should begin with "I." Such affirmations might include:

I am beautiful.
I am relaxed and rested.
I am a good mother/father/spouse.

Practice giving yourself affirmations and you may be surprised at how effective they can be at replacing self-deprecating thinking with positive personal images.

▼▼▼▼▼▼▼▼▼▼▼▼▼▼▼▼▼▼▼▼▼▼▼▼

DR. WALKER: ON A PERSONAL NOTE

We all come across situations in our lives that are unfair, situations that make us angry. In many cases, we experience anger, then find it difficult to let go; we carry around the anger long after the issue has passed.

I know this is true from personal experience. During my medical residency I felt I was unjustly treated by an attending physician. He said a number of rude and unbelievable things to me over the years. I felt anger at the time, and I held on to my anger against him for almost ten years.

Over time I realized that my anger was robbing my energy and affecting my relationships with new people. I developed a fear of reaching out and fully experiencing myself. I had to make a choice: I could either forgive him for those events or I could continue to punish myself by seeing myself as he did back then.

The decision was difficult for me because it meant that I had to give up my feelings of having been victimized by this person. I did some of the anger exercises we talk about here and I learned to forgive him—and myself—for the past. I began to see how my anger was limiting my life; I was able to call back my energy from the past situation so that I could live in the moment. I was able to see that in many ways the experience made me stronger. This was a tremendous blessing for me, and I wish the same for you.

WHEN STRESS RELIEF IS NOT ENOUGH

While the techniques described in this chapter can be very effective at easing stress and learning forgiveness, there are situations that require more dramatic steps. In some cases, the best way to deal with a situation is to remove yourself from it.

Consider the case of a forty-eight-year-old African American man we knew for almost ten years. He struggled with addiction to multiple medications and street drugs. He had chronic back and muscle pain; he suffered from panic attacks and was sometimes so afraid that he would not leave his house.

We talked for years about his plan for recovery, then about a year ago he took a bold step and moved out West. As part of his soul-searching mission, he went to an Indian reservation, where he was welcomed. There he discovered that he had a sense of humor; he found that people enjoyed being around him; and he found that his symptoms, addictions, and temptations did not bother him.

A few months later, he returned—and his pain promptly returned as well. His family and friends undermined him and diminished him by criticizing his dream. He realized that his body was talking to him; his body supported his dream and told him to go West. He left again—this time for good—when he realized that he had the courage required to become a success.

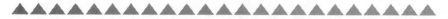

MIND-BODY STRESS-RELIEF TECHNIQUES

Understanding our anger and finding appropriate ways of expressing this powerful emotion can alleviate some of the stress in our lives, but it takes more than anger management to ease the physical symptoms of daily stress. No single stress-reduction technique works magically for everyone, but we recommend that almost all of our patients experiment with one or more stress-reduction techniques in an attempt to find one that works for them.

It's impossible to eliminate all sources of stress and negative emotions, but we can minimize the harmful effects of stress on our bodies. Just as your body can't tell the difference between the stress of a tiger attack and the stress of losing your job, your body can't tell whether the relaxation response was triggered by a change in circumstances or a change in your attitude. This can work to your advantage because you can learn to promote relaxation and reverse the stress response by using various mind-body techniques.

Studies have shown that people who practice relaxation exercises regularly have the ability to use mind-body techniques to voluntarily lower their blood pressure and heart rate, alter their brain wave activity, reduce blood sugar levels, and ease muscle tension. With practice, you too can use your mind to help overcome illness. The following techniques can help.

Biofeedback

Biofeedback involves training yourself to use your mind to voluntarily control the body's internal systems. The technique has been successfully used to treat shortness of breath due to congestive heart failure, to assist in stroke rehabilitation, to help diabetics lower their blood-glucose levels, to lower blood pressure, and to relieve incontinence, among other applications. It is also helpful in the treatment of insomnia and intestinal problems.

Almost anyone can learn biofeedback, but it takes practice. It's easy to get stressed out, but you can learn to relax and control the precise effect of mind over body. To learn the skill, you must be able to measure your physical state. To do this, electrodes are attached to various parts of your body to measure your heart rate, breathing, perspiration, pulse, blood pressure, temperature, muscle tension, and brainwave patterns. A small machine on the other end of the wires displays the data, usually in the form of pictures, graphic lines, or audible beeps. Using this information, you can literally watch yourself relax or grow more tense.

You can actually learn to control your body's internal processes by carefully studying the measurable changes in your body as you relax and change your thought patterns. Once you learn to adjust your physical state to promote relaxation, you can do it without all the equipment.

If you'd like to try biofeedback, ask your physician for a referral to an outpatient clinic or look for biofeedback centers listed in the phone book. Before making an appointment, ask about fees and whether or not the training will be covered by your health insurance plan. For a referral you can also contact the Association for Applied Psychophysiology and Biofeedback, 10200 W. 44th Avenue, Suite 304, Wheat Ridge, CO 80033, (303) 422-8436, or the Biofeedback Certification Institute of America, 10200 W. 44th Avenue, Suite 304, Wheat Ridge, CO 80033, (303) 420-2902.

Breathing

Deep breathing helps to relax the body and quiet the mind. Unfortunately, most people don't breathe right when stressed: Instead of inhaling deeply and drawing in plenty of oxygen, they take shallow, rapid, weak breaths, filling only the top part of the lungs. This so-called chest breathing, or thoracic breathing, fails to oxygenate the blood adequately, making it more difficult to manage stress, resulting in anxiety, panic attacks, depression, headaches, fatigue, and muscle tension, among other problems. Deep breathing sets forth an internal rhythm in the body, like the heartbeat, and it is useful in the treatment of all physical problems. (The entire body functions better when supplied with oxygen-rich blood.)

The alternative and preferred way of breathing is "abdominal breathing," or diaphragmatic breathing. This type of breathing draws air deeply into the lungs, allowing the chest to fill with air and the belly to rise and fall. Newborn babies and sleeping adults practice abdominal breathing, though most adults lapse into chest breathing during their waking hours.

To relieve stress, become aware of your breathing and inhale more fully; most people will immediately be able to feel the muscle tension and stress melt away in response to the improved oxygenation in your tissues. Concentrated, deep breathing can help calm you and relieve stress at any time and in any situation. Of course, don't overdo it or you will hyperventilate. If you experience shortness of breath, heart palpitations, or a feeling that you can't get enough air when practicing deep breathing, stop immediately and return to your regular breathing pattern.

Massage

Massage offers a hands-on way of reducing stress and promoting overall health. The technique—which involves the soothing touch of the muscles, soft tissues, and ligaments of the body—stimulates blood circulation, slows the heart rate, and lowers blood pressure. It also strengthens the immune system by stimulating the production of disease-fighting antibodies, and it releases toxins from the lymphatic system. Studies have found that massage reduces anxiety and stress-related hormones better than other muscle-relaxation techniques. And instead of making you feel drowsy, it can actually increase your alertness. Because of these health-promoting benefits, massage is useful in the treatment of almost every illness.

You can learn massage techniques yourself, either by checking out a book from a local library or by taking a class. You might also consider consulting a massage therapist, who should know a variety of techniques. Most states require licensing of massage therapists; if your state doesn't have licensing, look for a therapist with certification from a professional organization. For information on state licensing requirements and a list of certified massage therapists in your area, call the National Certification Board for Therapeutic Massage and Bodywork at (800) 296-0664. You can also contact the American Massage Therapy

Association, 820 Davis Street, Suite 100, Evanston, IL 60201, (708) 864-0123, or the American Oriental Bodywork Therapy Association, Glendale Executive Campus, 1000 White Horse Road, Vorhees, NJ 08043, (609) 782-1616.

Meditation

Though it comes in many different forms or traditions, meditation basically involves focusing your complete attention on one thing at a time. If you haven't tried it, meditation can be harder than it sounds: The mind tends to wander, and it can be a real challenge to maintain concentration when faced with a barrage of distracting thoughts.

Meditation relieves stress because it is impossible to feel tense or angry when your mind is focused somewhere else. You can't experience negative thoughts—or the physiological responses to those thoughts—if your mind is tuned in to a neutral stimulus. The quiet mind promotes overall health; meditation helps you stop wasting energy on negative thoughts.

Studies back up the idea that meditation promotes relaxation. Research done back in 1968 at Harvard Medical School found that when people practiced transcendental meditation (a type of mantra meditation) they showed physiological signs of deep relaxation: Their heart rate and breathing slowed, their oxygen consumption dropped by 20 percent, their skin resistance to electrical current increased, and their brainwave patterns showed greater alpha wave activity.

To experience the relaxing benefits of meditation, find a quiet place where you are not apt to be interrupted. If possible, sit in a firm chair with your back as straight as possible. If sitting is uncomfortable, lie down flat on your back on the ground. Your goal is to gain mastery over attention. Concentration is essential. Then try one of the three basic types of meditation:

- *Mantra meditation* involves repeating—either aloud or silently—a word (such as *peace* or *calm*), a syllable (such as *ommmm*), or a group of words (such as "I am safe" or "It's okay") each time you breathe out.

- *Gazing meditation* involves focusing both your attention and your gaze on an object such as a candle flame, a stone, or a flower. The object should be about one foot away from your face. Gaze at it rather than stare, keeping your eyes relaxed. Don't try to think about the object in words; just look at it without judgment.

- *Breathing meditation* involves focusing on the rise and fall of your breath. Draw a deep breath, focusing on the inhalation, the pause before you exhale, the exhalation, and the pause before you inhale. When you exhale, say to yourself "one." Each time you complete a breath and exhale, count again, one through four, then start over with one. The counting helps clear your mind of other thoughts.

No matter which type of meditation you choose, begin your session with a few minutes of deep breathing. When random thoughts enter your mind during your meditation time (as they almost certainly will), don't become anxious; just accept the thoughts and let them pass through your mind without notice or response. Start by meditating for five to ten minutes once or twice a day, then work up to fifteen to twenty minutes.

The process may seem deceptively simple. Once you have truly tried to quiet your mind, or to allow images to run through it without letting any particular one become distracting, you will understand why practice is necessary for success.

Numerous studies have demonstrated that meditation is psychologically and physiologically more refreshing and energy restoring than deep sleep. In fact, many meditators have reported that they required noticeably less sleep after they began meditating. Meditation is a profoundly regenerative process.

For more information on meditation, refer to books in the library or contact:

Cambridge Insight Meditation Center
331 Broadway
Cambridge, MA 02139
(617) 491-5070

Foundation for Human Understanding
P.O. Box 1009
Grants Pass, OR 97526
(503) 597-4360

The Mind-Body Medical Institute
New England Deaconess Hospital
Harvard Medical School
110 Francis Street, Suite 1A
Boston, MA 02215

The Stress Reduction Clinic
University of Massachusetts Medical Center
55 Lake Avenue, North
Worcester, MA 01655
(508) 856-2656

The Zen Center
300 Page Street
San Francisco, CA 94102
(415) 863-3136

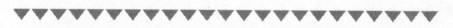

A WORD FROM DR. SINGLETON ON THE POWER OF PRAYER

I use prayer therapy often with my patients with excellent results. One experience that immediately comes to mind is the healing of a thirty-five-year-old woman with lupus, a degenerative disease of the connective tissues that rarely goes into remission. As part of my working with her, I asked if we could pray together. We asked God for healing, and from that moment on her condition dramatically improved. Over the next three months, she gradually went off her medication altogether. I had never seen anything like it.

Extensive research has documented the effectiveness of prayer in healing. One of the most inspiring books I've read on prayer is

Healing Words by Larry Dossey, M.D. One of the studies described in the book involves the effect of prayer on patients in the coronary care unit at San Francisco General Hospital. A computer assigned 393 patients to either a prayer group or a nonprayer group; a group of Christians were given the first name and a general description of the people in the prayed-for group, and they were asked to pray for them at least once a day. (Neither the doctors nor the patients knew which patients were in which group.)

The results: Patients in the group that was prayed for were five times less likely to require antibiotics, three times less likely to have heart failure and fluid buildup in the lungs, and fewer of these patients died compared with the patients who were not prayed for. None of the members of the prayed-for group needed to have assisted breathing, while twelve of the non-prayed-for group did.

I recommend that people pray for themselves and have other people pray for them. I am a Christian physician; I pray to a Christian God. This is my personal belief system, but the evidence suggests that prayer heals regardless of what God you worship. It appears that the healing comes from the power of the loving thoughts or positive intentions toward another person or toward oneself. To open your heart in prayer is to open yourself up to healing.

▲▲▲▲▲▲▲▲▲▲▲▲▲▲▲▲▲▲▲▲▲▲▲▲▲▲▲▲▲▲

Progressive Relaxation

Progressive relaxation can produce a profound feeling of calm as you systematically remove stress from your body. You can use the technique to retrain your nervous system and ease muscle spasms associated with asthma and irritable bowel syndrome.

Start by lying on your back on the floor with your legs flat and your arms loose at your sides. Close your eyes and breathe deeply. Once you are reasonably calm, begin to systematically tense and relax every muscle in your body. Start with your feet: Tense the muscles in your feet for thirty seconds or so, then relax, allowing your feet to feel heavy and relaxed. Then move on to your calves, thighs, abdomen, buttocks, hands, forearms, upper arms, shoulders, and face. When you finish, your muscles should feel soothed and relaxed. Lie quietly and enjoy the feeling of complete relaxation.

Visualization

To relieve stress, use your imagination. Visualization—also known as guided imagery—builds on the idea that you are what you think you are; where the mind goes, the body will follow. If you think anxious thoughts, your muscles will grow tense; if you think sad thoughts, your brain biochemistry will change and you will become unhappy. And, more important, if you think soothing, positive thoughts, you will relax and develop a more positive outlook. This technique is an important tool in the treatment of any illness or medical problem, since it can be used to set a direction for the healing process.

To experience the relaxation of visualization, sit down in a comfortable position or lie on the floor in a quiet, dimly lit room. Tense all of your muscles at once and hold for thirty seconds. Relax every muscle and allow all the tension to drain from your body. Continue to inhale and exhale slowly and fully.

Once your muscles have relaxed, you can begin the visualization or imagery. First, concentrate on your breathing, feeling the regular rhythm of each breath and clearing your mind of all thoughts. Then imagine that you are in a peaceful setting, such as lying in the warm sun on a sandy beach or strolling down a country road on a cool October afternoon. Get all of your senses involved in your image: Smell the ocean mist; hear the leaves crunch under your feet. The more specific your fantasy, the more real it will seem. And the more real it seems, the more you will relax. Enjoy this "escape" for about twenty minutes. When you return to your body and get on with the challenges of the day, you will probably feel much more relaxed and refreshed.

You can also use guided imagery to visualize changes in your physical state. For example, if you have asthma, you might imagine your lung passages opening up, or if you have arthritis, you might visualize your muscles relaxing and your joints smoothly gliding through a full range of motion. The technique has been shown to help in the treatment of chronic pain, allergies, high blood pressure, and stress-related health problems. Many of the health benefits are directly related to the link between visualization and relaxation.

However, guided imagery has also been used in the treatment of cancer (patients visualize powerful immune system cells consuming and destroying cancer cells). While no well-controlled study has been conducted to prove the direct impact of guided imagery on cancer, studies have shown that the technique helps to ease anxiety and pain, and to increase a patient's tolerance of chemotherapy and radiation treatment.

For more information on visualization, contact the Mind-Body Medical Institute, New England Deaconess Hospital, Harvard Medical School, 110 Francis Street, Suite 1A, Boston, MA 02215, (617) 632-9530, or The Academy for Guided Imagery, P.O. Box 2070, Mill Valley, CA 94942, (800) 726-2070.

Yoga

Yoga promotes relaxation while at the same time strengthening and stretching the muscles. It works to improve the functioning of the lymphatic system, realigns the energetic circulation in the body, and reduces waste from muscle tension. These health-promoting benefits make Yoga good for preventing illness as well as for healing the system as a whole.

Yoga combines deep breathing with systematically moving the body into a series of postures, or positions. It can be very gentle and non-competitive, making it an ideal exercise for people who have grown out of shape over the years. But some Yoga postures require significant endurance, strength, and flexibility. Since it works every muscle group, weaknesses can be identified easily, allowing you to target areas that may need special attention. If you have not exercised in a while, be sure to choose a class (or positions) for the beginner.

For background on Yoga postures and practicing the technique, check out a book or video on Yoga from your local library or take a class at a local "Y" or recreation facility. Look in the Yellow Pages under Yoga;

tune into PBS for a nationally syndicated show or rent a video. Or contact the Integral Yoga Institute, 227 West 13th Street, New York, NY 10011, (212) 929-0586.

RELIEVING STRESS WITH HERBS

Herbs can play an important role in stress management, especially when used in conjunction with mind-body techniques. (For specific information on using herbs, see Chapter 2, "East Meets West," page 21.)

Herbs for Daily Mild Stress

If you know that you're headed for a prolonged period of low-grade stress, prepare yourself by using these relaxing herbs to soothe your frazzled nerves. Known as nervine relaxants, these herbs can be used regularly as gentle soothing remedies. They include:

Balm (*Melissa officinalis*)
Chamomile (*Matricaria recutita*)
Kava kava (*Piper methysticum*)
Lavender (*Lavandula spp.*)
Linden (*Tilia spp.*)
Mugwort (*Artemisia vulgaris*)
Oats (*Avena sativa*)
Skullcap (*Scutellaria spp.*)
Vervain (*Verbena officinalis*)
Wood betony (*Stachys betonica*)

They can be used as teas, cold drinks, or infused in massage oil. They also make a relaxing footbath or an aromatic full bath. For information on making an herbal preparation, see Chapter 2, "East Meets West," page 21. If you use a commercial preparation, follow the package directions.

Herbs for Long-standing Stress

These herbs can be used for chronic stress:

> Ginseng *(Panax spp.)*
> Siberian ginseng *(Eleutherococcus senticosus)*

Herbs for Short-term Severe Stress

When your life feels out of control and you are under severe pressure, look for herbal relief. These herbs can help take the edge off the trauma, but they won't eliminate it altogether. Add the following to the list of herbs above:

> Passion flower *(Passiflora incarnata)*
> Valerian *(Valeriana officinalis)*
> Wild lettuce *(Lactuca virosa)*

Herb for Depression

When the stress of daily life has turned to depression, Saint-John's-wort *(Hypericum perforatum)* can help lift your spirits.

The Doctors' Antistress Tonic

Skullcap *(Scutellaria laterifolia)*	2 parts
Valerian *(Valeriana officinalis)*	2 parts
Oats *(Avena sativa)*	1 part

Mix the herbs using the proportions listed above. Prepare a tincture; take 1 teaspoon of it as needed. (For more information on using herbs, see pages 21, 315.)

STRESS AND AROMATHERAPY

A warm bath can be a stress buster after a trying day—and it can be even more effective when you add essential oils to take advantage of their soothing aroma. Use six to eight drops of your favorite formula or oil. You may also make up a massage oil, which can double as a body rub to put on before going to work. You can also use it in the shower in the morning.

Floral Garden

10 drops	lavender
10 drops	geranium
10 drops	palma rosa

Add the oils to 40 milliliters of a carrier oil, such as almond or jojoba.

Citrus Lovely

15 drops	clary-sage
10 drops	lemon
5 drops	lavender

Add the oils to 40 milliliters of a carrier oil, such as almond or jojoba.

Sunshine in the Morning

15 drops	marjoram
10 drops	lemon
5 drops	chamomile Roman

Add the oils to 40 milliliters of a carrier oil, such as almond or jojoba.

You can also make your own synergistic blends. Use the oils either singly or in a blend of up to three.

- Oils for *relaxation* include clary-sage, chamomile, cypress, geranium, lavender, lemon, marjoram, neroli, nutmeg, orange blossom, pettigraine, rose, sandalwood, and vetiver.

- *Hypnotic* (or *heavily sedative*) oils include carnation, hop, hyacinth, jasmine, jonquil, michela alba, narcissus, osmanthus, rose maroc, tonka bean, valerian, and vanilla.

- *Performance stress* oils (which can be effective before stressful one-time events, such as making a speech or taking an exam) include benzoin, bergamot, clary-sage, coriander, ginger, grapefruit, lemon, neroli, palma rosa, rose, and rosemary.

Use the oils in a bath or shower before the event, inhaling deeply while you do so. Or add a drop to a tissue to take with you and inhale when needed. Use four to six drops in the bath or three drops on a washcloth in the shower. Always be sure to mix the oils into the water with your hand before getting into the tub. Essential oils are highly concentrated and have been known to "burn" the skin if not adequately diluted.

NOTE: Do not use essential oils if you are pregnant.

▼▼▼▼▼▼▼▼▼▼▼▼▼▼▼▼▼▼▼▼▼▼▼▼▼▼

OUR HERITAGE OF HEALING

To relieve stress and to promote healing, some of our African ancestors use aromatics during the bathing process, but not in the same way we use essential oils and aromatics in our practice today. In the Sudan, some people clean themselves using what is essentially a steam bath. They dig a hole in the ground and place in it a pot containing a strong-smelling "wood of the tulloch." The "bather" sits over the pot, covered by a wool blanket, for ten minutes or so. The intense perspiration allows toxins to escape through the skin; the aromatic quality of the smoke invigorates the body. Different woods can be used for fumigations in the treatment of disease.

▲▲▲▲▲▲▲▲▲▲▲▲▲▲▲▲▲▲▲▲▲▲▲▲▲

TAKE TIME OUT FOR AN ACUPRESSURE MOMENT

Stress relief is right at your fingertips. Acupressure can be used to help the body relax and let go of anger and negative emotions. For more information on acupressure and illustrations of the points, see Chapter 2, "East Meets West," pages 29–37. The following five acupressure points are among the most powerful for relaxation and stress relief:

- **Bladder 10** (Heavenly Pillar). This point is located one finger width below the base of the skull on the ropy muscles one-half inch outside the spine. It is used to relieve stress, fatigue, insomnia, eyestrain, stiff necks, swollen eyes, and sore throats.

- **Triple Warmer 15** (Heavenly Rejuvenation). Place your fingers on the shoulders, midway between the base of the neck and the outside of the shoulders, one-half inch below the top of the shoulders. This point is used to relieve nervous tension and stiff necks.

- **Governing Vessel 24.5** (Third Eye Point). This point is located directly between the eyebrows in the ridge where the bridge of the nose meets the forehead. It is used to calm the body and relieve nervousness.

- **Conception Vessel 17** (Sea of Tranquillity). To locate this point, place your fingers on the center of the breastbone three thumb widths up from the base of the bone. This point relieves nervousness, anxiety, chest tension, heartache, depression, and other emotional imbalances.

- **Heart 7** (Spirit Gate). This point is located on the little finger side of the forearm at the crease of the wrist. It relieves fear, nervousness, anxiety, forgetfulness, and other emotional imbalances.

▼▼▼▼▼▼▼▼▼▼▼▼▼▼▼▼▼▼▼▼▼▼▼▼▼

LIFE SKILLS FOR STRESS AVOIDANCE

Better than managing stress is avoiding it altogether. The following communication skills can help:

- *Explore the ways you manage conflict.* When we experience conflict with another person, we have a chance to argue and blame—or to see the situation as an opportunity for individual growth. If you choose personal growth, you can:

  —take responsibility for your emotional reaction to the situation

  —avoid blaming the other person or defending yourself

  Before responding to a person when you are engaged in conflict, take a moment to calm yourself, to establish a clear and positive intention, and to look for a creative solution. Remember that you are talking to another valuable human being; each conflict can be seen as a chance to build your relationship with the other person and with yourself.

- *Express the positive.* Too often too many of us express criticism and negative feelings without hesitation, but hold back when it comes to telling someone something positive and loving. The more you express the positive, the more you get into the habit of looking for—and recognizing—the positive in other people. This affirming habit will create a positive focus for your relationships and start to change your own mind-body healing pattern.

- *Be open to criticism.* When someone gives us criticism (or feedback), we can either respond defensively or use the information as an opportunity for learning. The more open we are to receiving feedback and assessing its merits, the more we will grow and learn about ourselves. Of course, that doesn't mean we need to accept and internalize unwarranted or hostile criticism, but we will benefit if we are open to hearing the feedback (without the judgment), and we can then assess its value. We can use the information to ask ourselves, Are my actions working? Is there a way I can change what I'm doing and become more effective? Is there a pattern to my behavior that I could consider changing? If the feedback is mixed with anger, try to listen to the words and disregard the negative energy associated with those words.

- *Give loving feedback.* Accurate, caring, specific feedback can be used to help someone else recognize ways that they might change their behavior or attitudes. For feedback to be effective, it must be honest and loving. Before speaking, ask the person's permission: "I would like to offer some feedback. Would you be open to that?" If the person says, "No," then don't give any feedback.

- *Make sure your message has been heard.* Effective communication requires that people hear both the words we say and the meaning behind those words. Miscommunication often occurs when we assume that someone has heard and understood our message. Rather than relying on assumptions, periodically check to be sure your message has been sent and accurately received. This "perception checking" has nothing to do with your point of view or your opinion; it has to do with clarity. "I heard you say . . . . ; is that accurate?" If there was any confusion, it gives both parties a chance to clarify their message.

- *Ask open-ended questions.* To get to know someone, ask questions that invite them to open up. In other words, don't ask yes-no questions. Don't ask, "Is your job going well?" (Possible answer: Yes.) Instead ask, "What has been happening at your job?" (This requires some detail in the response.)

▲▲▲▲▲▲▲▲▲▲▲▲▲▲▲▲▲▲▲▲▲▲▲▲▲▲▲▲

5

▼

Back into Balance

A Customized Diet for African Americans

Let your food be your medicine.
—HIPPOCRATES

Among the Kung Bushmen of northwest Botswana, high blood pressure, high cholesterol levels, and obesity are unknown. In fact, the blood cholesterol levels of the Bushmen are among the lowest of any people in the world.

A well-balanced diet undoubtedly contributes to the outstanding overall health of these native people. So what are they eating? The most significant single food in the Bushman diet is the mongongo nut, which is a good source of protein and linoleic acid. They also eat a variety of vegetables and they occasionally indulge in wild honey, but they eat no other form of concentrated sugar. They do eat meat—primarily wild hares and other small animals—but only intermittently.

In contrast, consider the diet of the typical African American today. We eat a lot of starchy, fatty, sugary foods that increase insulin levels and contribute to inflammation. We consume animal fats, fried foods, refined sugars and flours, and processed foods with lots of additives. Few of us eat healthy amounts of fruits and vegetables. Our poor diet has triggered a number of significant health problems, including obesity, heart disease, and cancer, among others.

While such an unbalanced diet is unhealthy for people of any race, it can be particularly hazardous for African Americans. We have inherited from our ancestors a distinctive metabolic type, and we need to eat a diet that reflects our physical heritage. For too long we have been trapped in the conventional one-size-fits-all approach to diet, but no single diet is right for everyone. This chapter can help you customize a diet plan that meets the nutritional needs for your individual genetic makeup.

The dietary recommendations we make in this chapter have proved helpful with many of our African American patients. The diet is designed for overall good health, not for weight loss. If you need to lose weight, see Chapter 7, "Reshaping Your Body: Developing a Strategy for Weight Control," page 115.

OUR METABOLIC INHERITANCE

As African Americans, we have bodies that function best when fueled by the same foods as those consumed by our ancestors, hunter-gatherers who ate lean red meat and foods high in protein. These distant relatives consumed few dairy products or grains, but they did eat a lot of high-fiber vegetables and fruits. In fact, the average stool volume among our African ancestors was *nine times* what it is today in the United States, a reflection of the high fiber content of their diet.

To be healthy, we need not re-create this native diet, but we will be well served if we try to learn from it. Even among African Americans, no single diet formula will work for everyone. A number of factors contribute to individual metabolism, including genetic history, exercise, and the foods you eat. Just as some engines run on 89-octane fuel and others on diesel, we must learn which type of fuel our bodies require for optimal performance.

One marker for this metabolic pattern is blood type. Most African Americans have blood type O. Unless you're donating blood or facing a blood transfusion you may assume that your blood type makes little difference in your daily life, but recent research indicates that your blood type may have a critical bearing on your metabolism and on the foods you should—and shouldn't—eat.

Our years of experience support the conclusion that African Americans have unique nutritional needs. After considering the eating habits of our patients over the years, we have come up with this simple list of dietary guidelines for African Americans.

- *African Americans need to eat more protein than most diets recommend.* Our African ancestors ate a diet high in plant-based proteins, such as nuts, and ultralean meat from wild animals. (The meat from wild animals is far leaner than even the leanest cuts of meat from livestock bred for human consumption.) Red meat was usually eaten as part of religious rites and ceremonies. Our bodies crave protein; most African Americans will thrive on a diet high in plant-based protein.

- *African Americans should avoid eating excessive amounts of grains, especially wheat.* Our distant relatives did not eat grains as a dietary staple, and their bodies were ill suited for digesting these foods. Grains are very common in the typical American diet; it comes as no surprise that many African Americans have trouble digesting them, leading to gastrointestinal distress and skin problems. In addition, we have found that grains contribute to weight gain among African Americans. If you need to reduce, you may be able to lose weight—even if you don't cut calories—by cutting grain-based products from your diet.

- *African Americans should minimize their consumption of animal fats.* Our ancestors ate plant-based fats, but little saturated animal fat. All fats are not created equal. Animal fats, saturated fats, oxidized fats, and cholesterol can be toxic to the body, but plant-based fats and essential fatty acids (which can be found in certain fish) can promote health by helping our bodies make hormones and reduce inflammation. Fat should not be feared. Instead, you need to avoid most animal fats and fried foods, while continuing to eat plant-based fats, such as soy products, olive oil, and avocados.

- *African Americans should avoid dairy products.* As hunter-gatherers, our ancestors consumed little or no lactose in their diets. As a result, many African Americans lack the enzyme necessary to break down lactose (milk sugar). If you are lactose intolerant or experience gastrointestinal distress after eating dairy products (including cheese and milk), then avoid eating them whenever possible. Problems with lactose intolerance have become more prevalent in the last few decades because the pasteurization process kills many of the natural enzymes that assist with digestion.

- *African Americans should limit their intake of refined carbohydrates (sugars).* Our African ancestors ate an abundant supply of complex carbohydrates—especially fruits and vegetables—but they did not eat refined carbohydrates, such as refined sugar. In the body, refined sugar stimulates the pancreas to produce insulin, which is needed for the metabolism of sugar. African Americans have a high rate of insulin-dependent diabetes, which may be a consequence of our difficulty metabolizing refined carbohydrates.

WHAT YOU SHOULD EAT:
A BALANCED DIET FOR AFRICAN AMERICANS

African Americans need to rebalance their diets by taking into account their metabolic inheritance. When we start talking about diets with many of our patients, they worry that eating right will restrict their freedom to make food choices, or that we will require complex formulas for calculating calories or keeping track of blocks of protein, fat, and carbohydrates. In reality, eating a balanced diet is just as easy as eating an unbalanced diet; all you need to do is to become familiar with the foods that should be the foundation of your diet and choose those foods at most of your meals.

The following lists of foods can serve as the cornerstone of your daily diet. They will provide balanced nutrition and they will also help your body maintain superior metabolic and hormone balance. You can, of course, modify this cornerstone diet based on your own unique needs, but you should strive to eat as many of your foods from these lists as possible.

Experiment with your diet, using the foods on these lists as a guide. Your body will give you feedback if it doesn't feel right. You should feel satisfied for four or five hours after eating; if you feel hungry or fatigued one or two hours after a meal, you may need to cut back on the carbohydrates and add protein.

Give your body time to adjust to your new eating habits; you will be quite pleased with the positive feelings you will encounter as your body becomes reconciled to your new diet. For example, if you're used to eating a breakfast high in simple carbohydrates (such as orange juice and a bagel) and you switch to a complex carbohydrate meal (such as oatmeal and grapefruit juice), you will experience fluctuations in your energy levels during the morning (which reflects your blood sugar levels). Also, over a period of several weeks, you will find your food cravings and desires will change, and sticking to the foundation diet will be both simple and satisfying.

The Primary Foods: Fruits and Vegetables

These foods are the backbone of a healthy diet. They are low in calories and allergenic substances and high in fiber and in vitamins, minerals, antioxidants, and phytonutrients.

apples	artichokes
bean sprouts	beets
broccoli	Brussels sprouts
cabbage	cauliflower
celery	cherries
Chinese cabbage	cucumbers
dandelion greens	dark green lettuce
eggplant	grapefruit
grapes	green beans
green peppers	kale
mushrooms	mustard greens
onions	parsley
peaches	pears
plums	spinach
tomatoes	turnip greens
watercress	zucchini

Others: Most fruits and vegetables can be added to the list, but strive to eat those with a low glycemic index. (For more information on the glycemic index, see page 94.)

Complex Carbohydrates

Carbohydrates should be in as natural a form as possible to preserve the fiber and micronutrients found in the whole food.

barley

brown rice

cracked wheat berries

Great Northern beans

legumes

lima beans

oats and oatmeal

pumpkins

split peas

sweet potatoes

whole grain rye bread

yams

a limited amount of honey and
    blackstrap molasses for sweetening

black-eyed peas

cracked rye berries

garbanzo beans

kidney beans

lentils

millet

potatoes (never fried)

soy beans

sprouted grain bread

wheat germ

whole rye flakes

Others: You can add other complex carbohydrates to the list, but strive to eat those with a low glycemic index. (For more information on the glycemic index, see page 94.)

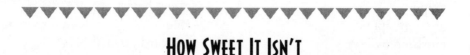

How Sweet It Isn't

You may have noticed that this list includes very few sugars and sweets. We have found that few African Americans do well with sugars and simple carbohydrates (remember, that African Bushmen ate honey only once in a while). With most of our patients, sweets raise the blood sugar levels and disrupt the body's delicate bacterial balance; the fungus and pathological bacteria in the gut feast on the excess sugar, throwing off the flora in the intestinal tract. You must look carefully at the ingredients in the foods you eat, since corn syrup is added to an enormous number of processed foods. You should always avoid refined cane (white) sugar; this highly processed sweetener is devoid of nutrition—though it can raise blood sugar levels and promote the growth of yeast in the body.

You may also have noted that the list included some grains and not others. As mentioned on page 87, African Americans often have difficulty digesting many grains. If you have trouble metabolizing wheat, corn, and other common grains, consider switching to rye, which is high in protein and easier to digest than other grains. If you love pasta, look for those made from artichokes, spinach, or other vegetables, and limit your pasta meals to two or three times a week.

▲▲▲▲▲▲▲▲▲▲▲▲▲▲▲▲▲▲▲▲▲▲▲▲▲▲▲▲

Proteins and Fats

Protein and fats are essential for balanced nutrition. Emphasize vegetable protein over animal protein, and avoid margarine, fried foods, and heated oils.

almonds	avocados
cashews	codfish
haddock	lean meats (except pork)
macadamia nuts	mackerel
olives and olive oil	peanuts
poultry (without the skin)	pumpkin seeds
salmon	soybeans
sunflower seeds	tofu
trout	tuna

Others: Additional proteins and fats can be added to the list, but you should avoid animal fats.

▼▼▼▼▼▼▼▼▼▼▼▼▼▼▼▼▼▼▼▼▼▼

CHOOSING WISELY WHEN CHOOSING PROTEINS

- We recommend that African Americans consume most of their protein in the form of nuts, seeds, avocados, and other plant sources. Some lean red meat can be helpful to some people, but it should be limited to two or three servings per week.

- Look for cold-pressed extra virgin olive oil. Cold-pressed oils have not been heated, so there is less oxidation than occurs in oils that have been extracted using heat and chemical solvents.

- Avoid pork, cured meats, or organ meats. These meats are difficult for the body to metabolize and should be eaten sparingly, if at all. As a rule of thumb, never consume more animal protein than you can fit on the palm of your hand. And when you do eat meat, look for range-fed animals, which should be free of antibiotics and hormones.

- Some people do well with small amounts of red meat; others do not. Talk to your doctor about the use of lean meats or experiment with your diet by adding small servings of lean red meat, then carefully assessing how you feel after eating these foods.

- Dairy foods can be high in protein, but as mentioned on pages 87–88, many African Americans experience symptoms of lactose intolerance (gas, bloating, and diarrhea) after consuming them. It is important to limit your intake of dairy foods even if you're not lactose intolerant in order to prevent the formation of allergies. If you do drink milk, instead of cow's milk, try goat's milk (which more closely resembles human breast milk), soy milk, almond milk, or oat milk. You might also want to eliminate dairy foods if you have a problem with eczema or other skin conditions, which can be triggered by lactose intolerance. We see a lot of dairy intolerance in our patients with eczema and other skin conditions. Once we tell them to cut the dairy out of their diet, their skin often clears up without the use of harsh chemicals.

▲▲▲▲▲▲▲▲▲▲▲▲▲▲▲▲▲▲▲▲▲▲▲▲▲

HOW MUCH TO EAT: CUSTOMIZING THE DIET TO MEET YOUR NEEDS

While fruits and vegetables, complex carbohydrates, proteins, and fats make up every diet, different people have different dietary needs and should eat different proportions of the foods from the lists above. We use an individual's triglyceride level as a guide to making dietary recommendations. (To find out your triglyceride level, ask your doctor to perform the simple blood test.)

In general, as your triglyceride levels go up, you should scale back on complex carbohydrates and increase your consumption of proteins. Following are the guidelines we use:

- If your triglyceride level is less than 70, you should eat in the following proportions:

  40 percent of calories from fruits and vegetables
  20 percent of calories from complex carbohydrates
  20 percent of calories from protein
  20 percent of calories from fat

- If your triglyceride level is 70 to 140, you should eat in the following proportions:

  40 percent of calories from fruits and vegetables
  10 percent of calories from complex carbohydrates
  30 percent of calories from protein
  20 percent of calories from fat

- If your triglyceride level is over 140, you should eat in the following proportions:

  50 percent of calories from fruits and vegetables

5 percent of calories from complex carbohydrates
30 percent of calories from protein
15 percent of calories from fat

Even with the proportions listed above, you don't need to be a slave to measuring and recording the foods you eat. Instead, we recommend that you try to keep your plate proportioned. In other words, try to have most of the foods on your plate come from these core lists, and try to have the food quantities in the amounts listed above.

UNDERSTANDING THE GLYCEMIC INDEX

What makes one food "better" for you than another? Different foods contain different nutrients, of course, but they are also metabolized differently. For example, all carbohydrates contain four calories per gram, but they can have wildly different effects on the body's blood sugar levels.

You can use a food's "glycemic index" to measure its effect on blood sugar levels and to help you make wise food choices. The glycemic index is a measurement used to compare how high and how fast the blood sugar is raised by certain carbohydrate foods. The lower the glycemic index, the lesser the impact a food will have on the blood sugar levels. This issue is especially important for African Americans because we have inherited a propensity toward developing diabetes, a disease directly affecting the metabolism of carbohydrates and sugars.

▼▼▼▼▼▼▼▼▼▼▼▼▼▼▼▼▼▼▼▼▼▼▼▼

KNOW YOUR CARBOHYDRATES

All carbohydrates are created by photosynthesis in plants, but they have very different structures. Carbohydrates can be:

- simple sugars (such as those in honey and fruits)

- multiple sugars (such as table sugar and malt sugar)

- starches or complex carbohydrates (including vegetables, such as carrots, potatoes, and yams; and whole grains, such as rice, corn, and wheat)

- fiber (cellulose or hemicellulose, the indigestible roughage found in unprocessed carbohydrate-containing foods)

Whatever the form, all carbohydrates provide quick energy for the body and can be easily converted by the body to glucose.

▲▲▲▲▲▲▲▲▲▲▲▲▲▲▲▲▲▲▲▲▲▲▲▲▲

The foods listed above as part of the balanced diet for African Americans are low-glycemic foods. For example, the list of fruits includes grapes, grapefruits, and apples (which have a low glycemic index), but not bananas (which have a high glycemic index). That doesn't mean you must swear off bananas forever, but only that you should make low-glycemic fruits the mainstay of the fruit portion of your diet.

In the body, high-glycemic carbohydrates head straight for the liver, where they are broken down into glucose or sugar. The pancreas then kicks into gear, producing insulin to move the sugar into the cells. The sugar can be used for energy (causing the so-called sugar rush). Both the liver and the muscles store as much glucose as they can (in the form of glycogen), but when they have been saturated, the rest of the calories get tucked away as fat.

The glycemic index helps explain why so many weight-loss diets fail. Dieters restrict their calories and fat consumption, but they continue to eat foods high on the glycemic index scale. A lot of our patients come in and complain, "I don't know why I can't lose weight; I'm starving all the time." When asked, "What do you eat?" they respond, "All I had to eat for breakfast was a bagel and orange juice. For lunch I had a salad, a rice cake, and a baked potato, and for dinner I had some pasta."

It's no wonder these folks can't lose weight (and it's only by depriving themselves of an adequate caloric intake that they avoid putting on the pounds). These diligent dieters have wisely chosen low-fat foods, but they have foolishly selected high-glycemic foods.

In order to keep your body in balance (and to lose weight) you need to eliminate high-glycemic foods. If you eat foods that are starchy or relatively high on the glycemic scale, you need to balance them in a 1:3 ratio with green leafy vegetables and low-glycemic foods. When comparing French bread and a candy bar, many people assume the candy would trigger a faster and stronger glycemic reaction. However, because of the fat in the candy bar, it has a less dramatic impact on insulin levels than the bread.

▼▼▼▼▼▼▼▼▼▼▼▼▼▼▼▼▼▼▼▼▼▼▼▼▼▼

THE GLYCEMIC INDEX

The following chart divides common carbohydrates into categories based on their glycemic index. (The list is far from comprehensive; it includes a sampling of the foods that have been tested in a clinical setting.) Whenever possible, eat foods from the low or very low glycemic food lists. Foods that are low on the glycemic index tend not to raise blood sugar levels and have a minimal insulin response. Of course, high-glycemic foods can be good sources of nutrition, but they should not be used in excess.

Simple Sugars

Fructose	20
Sucrose	59
Honey	87
Glucose	100

Fruits

Apples	39
Oranges	40
Orange juice	48
Bananas	62
Raisins	64

Starchy Vegetables

Sweet potatoes	48
Yams	51

Beets	64
White potatoes	70
Instant potatoes	80
Carrots	92
Parsnips	97

Dairy Products

Skim milk	32
Whole milk	34
Ice cream	36
Yogurt	36

Legumes

Soybeans	15
Lentils	29
Kidney beans	29
Black-eyed peas	33
Garbanzo beans	36
Lima beans	36
Baked beans	40
Frozen peas	51

Pasta, Corn, Rice, Bread

Whole wheat pasta	42
White pasta	50
Sweet corn	59
Brown rice	66
White bread	69
Whole wheat bread	72
White rice	72

Breakfast Cereals

Oatmeal	49
All-bran	51
Shredded wheat	67
Cornflakes	80

Miscellaneous

Peanuts	13
Sausages	28
Tomato soup	38
Potato chips	51
Mars bar	68

▲▲▲▲▲▲▲▲▲▲▲▲▲▲▲▲▲▲▲▲▲▲▲▲▲▲▲

THE ULTIMATE TEST OF ANY DIET: HOW IT MAKES YOU FEEL

We cannot eat an unbalanced diet for a prolonged period of time without our bodies rebelling and becoming sick. Fortunately, switching to a balanced diet consisting of low-glycemic foods can help the body heal itself and remain healthy.

Food can be good medicine. A dramatic example involves a forty-one-year-old woman who came to the office in the spring of 1986 because she suffered from inflammatory bowel disease and Crohn's disease. For more than four years she had experienced unceasing diarrhea and her condition had deteriorated, despite prolonged treatment with steroids and an operation to remove part of her small bowel.

She came to the office with the attitude "Nothing else has worked, so let's see what you can do." We put her on a no-sugar, low-wheat diet, and gave her supplements of goldenseal, ginger, and acidophilus. Within six weeks her condition had reversed itself; she has remained symptom-free for more than a decade. Though conventional treatment for such digestive disorders often fails, in our practices we have found that inflammatory bowel disease is very often curable by making dietary changes.

▼▼▼▼▼▼▼▼▼▼▼▼▼▼▼▼▼▼▼▼▼▼▼▼

THE DANGERS OF MSG

African Americans tend to be much more sensitive to the harmful effect of monosodium glutamate (MSG) than people of other races. MSG is often added to foods during processing to balance the flavors and prolong shelf life. It is also a by-product of food processing; at high temperatures, an amino acid known as glutamic acid breaks off from protein molecules and joins with sodium to form MSG. MSG is found in aged cheese, soy sauce, alcohol, peas, corn, mushrooms, and tomatoes.

In the body, MSG can cause chronic illness and nerve problems. Some patients complain of bloating, abdominal pain, anxiety, insomnia, and achy joints. People with asthma may find their symptoms get worse; congestion, hives, headache, and eczema are not uncommon.

Watch product labels carefully. MSG must be listed if it is used as an additive in its pure form. However, many food processors add it as hydrolyzed vegetable protein (which contains 10 to 40 percent MSG). The words *natural flavorings* can be another term used to disguise MSG.

▲▲▲▲▲▲▲▲▲▲▲▲▲▲▲▲▲▲▲▲▲▲▲▲▲▲▲▲▲

BEYOND PLANNING THE MENU

It's not just what you eat but how you eat that can affect your overall health. When we discuss diet and eating habits with our patients, we make a point to mention the following issues:

- **Chew your food well.** Sometimes our patients chuckle when we remind them to take time to chew their food thoroughly, but the truth is that many people don't chew their food well enough. Ideally, you should chew each bite of food twenty to thirty times. When you chew your food you mix the digestive enzymes in your mouth with the food you are eating; this helps to reduce the work your digestive system must do to break down the food. Chewing also helps break up the food, which reduces the amount of gas your body produces. When poorly chewed food particles make their way into the digestive system, the bacteria in your gut has a feast, releasing gas, which can cause problems with flatulence, cramping, and bloating.

- **Drink more water.** If your heart and kidneys work well, then water is the most important detoxifying agent we have. The body needs water to wash away toxins and speed their elimination. In addition to the eight to ten 8-ounce glasses of water you should be drinking each day, add an additional quart of water to facilitate detoxification. Consuming herbal teas and fruit and vegetable juices will also help.

  How much water is enough? My rule of thumb is to take your weight and divide it in half—that total is the ideal number of ounces of water you should drink each day. For example, if you weigh 150 pounds, you should consume 75 ounces of water each day.

  Drink a small amount of water with meals—about 4 to 6 ounces. This is enough to aid digestion, but not so much that you dilute the hydrochloric acid, which is needed for the digestion of the protein. Drink most of your fluids a half hour before meals and between meals.

  The best water has been filtered by reverse osmosis. (You can buy a reverse-osmosis unit, which filters water as it is pumped from the faucet, for about $500 to $1,000.) Don't drink distilled water, since its lack of minerals can draw other minerals from the body, leaving the system out of balance. Instead, drink filtered or purified water. Or, if you choose to drink distilled water, additional minerals need to be added to your diet.

- **Choose organic foods.** Whenever possible, buy fruits, vegetables, and meats that are certified organic. Organic foods should have less pesticide residue than nonorganic products. Look for the U.S. Department of Agriculture's organic label, which recently replaced the private certification network that was in place before 1998.

- **Avoid cooking with fats.** When most fats are heated, they become hydrogenated and they release harmful free radicals. Instead of oils, use water or broth for stir-fries; if you need oil for flavor, add a bit after cooking. If only heated oils will do, use olive oil or grapeseed oil; these oils can tolerate higher temperatures before they oxidize. Many African Americans need relatively liberal amounts of olive oil, so you don't need to restrict it entirely. Do not eat margarine; it contains damaging trans-fatty acids.

- **Don't cook in the microwave.** While you can use the microwave for heating water for herbal tea, avoid using it to prepare food because the oven heats the food to such a high temperature that it coagulates the proteins and the nutritional value of what you're eating is diminished. The heat also kills the natural enzymes in the foods that help with digestion. (Conventional ovens aren't as damaging to food because they heat more evenly; microwave ovens tend to overheat the food in certain spots.)

- **Stop eating at 7 P.M.** Give your pancreas a break; even your digestive system deserves a chance to rest and detoxify. Try to follow the 12 on/12 off rule of thumb: Eat from 7 A.M. to 7 P.M., and fast from 7 P.M. to 7 A.M. This shouldn't be a problem if you eat a diet high in low-glycemic foods and complex carbohydrates.

- **Eat it raw.** Nibble on raw, well-washed fruits and vegetables; when cooking foods, cook them for as short a time as possible. The longer you heat food, the more nutrients you lose. Whenever possible, broil, steam, or bake foods; frying adds fat and creates hazardous free radicals. If your system has trouble digesting raw foods, steam food for a few minutes.

- **Avoid artificial sweeteners.** In the body, aspartame is broken down into formaldehyde, which can be toxic to nerve tissue. Either use minimal amounts of honey or molasses—or better yet, retrain your palate to enjoy foods containing less sugar.

Cleansing Your System

Designing a Detoxification Program

When most people first learn about natural medicine, they get very excited about what they put into their bodies. Then, the more they understand about healing and wholeness, the more they realize that what comes *out* of their bodies is just as important as what goes *in*.

Detoxification involves cleansing the body of the harmful toxins that can cause many health problems, especially chronic degenerative diseases. Cleansing and the elimination of toxins are more important today than ever before, since we are exposed to many more chemicals and pollutants than we had been in the past. In addition, we voluntarily ingest many refined foods and sugars, as well as alcohol, nicotine, caffeine, and other substances that have toxic effects on the body.

Detoxification is particularly important to African Americans because we are exposed to more toxins than people of other races. We encounter pollutants and harmful chemicals on the job, in our communities, and even in our homes. A 1992 report by the U.S. Environmental Protection Agency concluded that African Americans and other people of color suffer disproportionately from exposure to dust, soot, carbon monoxide, ozone, sulfur, sulfur dioxide, lead, and emissions from hazardous-waste dumps.

We cannot poison our bodies and not expect to suffer a decline in overall health. The consequences of our toxic exposure include a higher incidence of cancer, cardiovascular disease, allergies, obesity, arthritis, and problems associated with a weakened immune system. African Americans tend to be exposed to more toxins than people of other races, which may help to account for our high rate of illness and premature death.

Fortunately, we can purify our bodies and begin a more healthful approach to life by engaging in a detoxification program. Detoxification gives our digestive organs a chance to rest, even if only for a day or two. The liver, kidneys, and gallbladder can better perform their vital functions when periodically given an opportunity for a little rest and relaxation.

Periodic cleansing can be used to improve health, treat disease, and prevent illness, in addition to stimulating creativity, spirituality, productivity, and mental clarity. While it can be difficult to make life-sustaining changes in our diet and health habits, detoxification can be an important first step toward a healthier way of life.

THE TRUTH ABOUT TOXINS

We can't avoid them: We are exposed to toxins with every breath we take, with every bite we eat, with every drink we swallow. And, as if that weren't enough, our bodies produce additional toxins and wastes as by-products of daily living. Our bodies churn out damaging free radicals as part of the normal metabolic process; naturally occurring bacteria and yeasts release toxins that can cause damage to the cells and cause health problems. Even mental stress and negative emotions can result in biochemical toxicity.

These toxic assaults can irritate or inflame the cells and tissues, making efficient elimination of toxins essential for good health. The potential damage of a toxic exposure depends on the amount, frequency, and potency of the toxin. Some toxins have immediate health-threatening effects, such as side effects caused by exposure to certain drugs or pesticides. Other toxins can build up in the body and cause a gradual decline in overall health in much the same way that exposure to saturated fats contributes to cardiovascular disease.

In large measure, our overall health depends on our body's ability to neutralize or eliminate these toxins. Our bodies do it all the time: The antioxidants in foods and supplements help to neutralize toxic free radicals; the liver filters out and alters substances that poison the body and releases them through the gastrointestinal tract; and the kidneys wash waste products out of the body via the urinary system. Even perspiration—whether caused by a jog around the block or a ten-minute session in a steamy sauna—helps release toxins from the body through the skin. Toxins can also be released through the sinuses and mucus membranes and for women through their menstrual cycle.

Of course, healthy bodies can handle exposures to many everyday toxins, but many people find that they can improve their health by periodically helping the body cleanse and detoxify itself. This is especially important for people exposed to daily emotional stress and those who challenge their systems by eating a diet that is high in saturated or animal fat, sugars, and refined flours. By following a program of detoxification, you can help your body eliminate the toxins that compromise your health.

DETOXIFY YOUR MIND

Before we discuss the importance of a nontoxic diet to purify the body, we must mention the importance of mental detoxification to purify the mind and spirit. We can improve our energy and outlook on life by cleansing the body of negative emotions and by focusing on forgiveness and healing rather than resentment and revenge. In many cases, the physical detoxification of the body can reinforce the mental detoxification of the spirit—just as purifying the mind can speed healing of the body and improve overall health.

This mind-body link was well known to our African ancestors. It was common practice for African medicine men or shamans to use drumming, fasting, and sweat baths as part of their healing process. Fasting not only detoxified the body, but it also helped to induce states of inspiration and to bring forth mystical experiences for the fasting tribal member.

While short-term periods of detoxification—several days to a week—can help improve your health and mood, longer-term or repeated detoxification sessions can help transform your life. Physically, detoxification can clear congestion and prevent disease, and emotionally, it can allow us to experience spiritual transformation and clarity of purpose in our lives. After detox, the body and spirit have been cleansed and made more open to the experience of love and hope and more prepared to replace negative lifestyle and eating habits with healthier ones.

THE DETOX DIET

When we mention detoxification to our patients, many of them think of a prolonged (and uncomfortable) water fast. While water fasting can be a powerful tool for detoxification, it is too extreme for many people and it is not the best choice for everyone.

Still, to clean out your body, you must clean up your diet. The better and more healthful your overall diet, the easier it will be to cleanse your system and keep it clean. If your diet has been less than ideal, do not despair: Instead, detoxify and then modify your diet on a more permanent basis.

In essence, any dietary changes you make that will speed elimination can be said to be part of a program of detoxification. You can start by making subtle changes in your approach to eating. There are several degrees of detoxification based on the extent of the dietary changes you are willing and able to make at the time.

- **Make simple changes in your eating habits.** You can begin the process of detoxification by switching from foods that are more congesting to those that are less so. Congesting foods contain more toxins and slow down the digestive system.

  MOST CONGESTING: Allergenic foods, organ meats, hydrogenated fats, other fats, fried foods, refined flour, meat and poultry, sugars
  MODERATELY CONGESTING: Milk, eggs, baked goods, wheat, rice, pasta
  LEAST CONGESTING: Beans, oats, millet, nuts, seeds, water, herbs, green vegetables, other vegetables, roots

- **Limit your diet to fresh fruits and vegetables and whole grains.** For a deeper level of detoxification, restrict your diet to these whole foods, either cooked or raw. Keep your food consumption at a 3:1 ratio, with three parts vegetables to one part fruit per meal. Avoid breads or baked goods and dairy products. This diet eliminates all animal products. The leafy green vegetables are very cleansing of the gastrointestinal system.

- **Eat only raw fruits and vegetables.** This diet takes the fruit-and-vegetable-and-grain diet one step farther, removing the grain and requiring that the foods be consumed raw. Maintain the three-to-one rule, choosing three servings of vegetables to one serving of fruit. Eating foods raw preserves the maximum levels of vitamins, minerals, and other nutrients.

▼▼▼▼▼▼▼▼▼▼▼▼▼▼▼▼▼▼▼▼▼▼▼▼▼

NOT ALL FRUITS ARE CREATED EQUAL

Fruits are high in fiber, but they also contain simple sugars that can convert to sugar very rapidly, in addition to encouraging certain problematic bacteria and yeast to grow in the gut. To minimize this problem, grapefruit, lemons, and limes are good choices, as are apples and grapes. The occasional kiwifruit for the treatment of constipation is okay. Bananas are very high in sugar and should be used sparingly by the average person.

▲▲▲▲▲▲▲▲▲▲▲▲▲▲▲▲▲▲▲▲▲▲▲▲▲

- **Drink only fruit and vegetable juices.** The next level of detoxification involves the exclusive use of juices, teas, and vegetable broths rather than whole foods. Fresh juices require minimal digestion, while providing essential nutrients. Miso, a form of fermented soybean, can also be eaten during this level of detoxification to encourage colon cleansing. We often recommend that our patients add spirulina, an algae powder available at health food stores, to their juices to avoid fatigue during a liquid juice fast. We believe juice fasts tend to be more healing than water fasts, since they flush the system while at the same time providing nutrients to nourish and rebuild the body.

- **Drink only water.** A water-only fast offers the oldest and most intense process of detoxification, but this type of fast leaves many people weak. However, fasting is one of the oldest forms of natural treatment, and it is a healing technique used by animals in the wild.

Our patients respond differently to detoxification. Some people find it invigorating—and others find it exhausting. We have had several patients who have been drained by the experience. It is like peeling an onion: As you release each layer, old symptoms may come forward in the process. They release on their own. If you have a detox reaction, usually backing off of the therapy and/or drinking a lot of water is helpful.

During the period of detoxification, most people can follow their normal routines, and many experience a boost in energy and creativity. However, some people do experience headaches, fatigue, and irritability. If you encounter any negative side effects during your detox, consider adding additional fruits, vegetables, and water.

If you're planning a liquid fast of more than three days, talk to a doctor or health care practitioner who can help you design a detoxification program suitable to your particular needs. If you want to experiment with detoxification on your own, start with minor modifications in your diet and progress to more intense changes over time. Try each phase for two or three days before moving on to the next.

Detoxification in general—and fasting in particular—may not be suitable for people who are underweight, sick, malnourished, or weak. Pregnant women and breast-feeding mothers should not attempt intense detoxification. People who tend to feel weak or fatigued during detox should consider cleansing for no more than three days.

During your detox program, consider taking certain dietary supplements to speed the cleansing and maintain nutrient balance. Many health food stores offer combination formulas designed for detoxification. A basic, low-dose multiple-vitamin, multiple-mineral supplement can provide the basic nutrients for daily living. Additional nutrients that can be helpful include fiber (to cleanse the colon), antioxidants (to neutralize free radicals and other toxins released during detox), and acidophilus bacteria (to neutralize toxins and stimulate the growth of healthy bacteria). After detoxification, consider supplementing your diet with the amino acid L-cysteine or N-acetyl glucosamine (to bind with mercury and other toxic heavy metals).

Since one of the goals of detoxification is colon cleaning, for two or three days you may want to take psyllium seeds or a mixture of psyllium seeds, aloe vera powder, and acidophilus culture, which will stimulate colon activity. (All of these ingredients are available at health food stores; follow package directions.) In the body, psyllium clears mucus from the intestines and draws toxins from the gastrointestinal tract. We often recommend that patients take one or two tablespoons of olive oil with the psyllium or fiber supplement to help bind the toxins. Some people are comfortable using water, herbal, or diluted coffee enemas to further cleanse the system.

An herbal treatment can also help stimulate detoxification. While hundreds of herbs can be used to cleanse the blood and tissues, we recommend that you look in the health food store for a commercially prepared detoxification formula that includes some of the following cleansing herbs:

aloe vera	beets*
burdock root	cayenne pepper
dandelion root	echinacea
garlic	gingerroot
goldenseal root*	licorice root
parsley root	red clover
sarsaparilla root	turmeric
yellow dock root	

▼▼▼▼▼▼▼▼▼▼▼▼▼▼▼▼▼▼▼▼▼▼▼▼

TOO MUCH OF A GOOD THING CAN BE DANGEROUS

If some is good, more is rarely better. It is possible to overdo detoxification. Overdetoxification or overelimination can cause people to lose essential nutrients and experience protein or vitamin and min-

---

* People with gallstones should take low doses of these herbs.

eral deficiencies. The overuse of fasting, laxatives, enemas, colonics, and diuretics can cause health problems. If you plan a detoxification program of more than one week, do so under the supervision of a physician or health care practitioner who has knowledge in this area.

▲▲▲▲▲▲▲▲▲▲▲▲▲▲▲▲▲▲▲▲▲▲▲▲▲▲▲▲▲

NOW, DETOXIFY THE REST OF YOUR LIFE

Dietary changes play a central role in detoxification, but lifestyle choices can be toxic, too. We ingest and expose ourselves to toxins in a number of ways throughout the day. During your detox—and as much as possible throughout your life—try to follow these tips on living the clean life:

Keep it natural. Try to avoid drugs (both prescription and over-the-counter drugs), which usually have some unwelcome side effects. Whenever possible, opt for herbs, homeopathic remedies, and nutrition supplements, which usually have fewer and less severe side effects. Massage therapy, acupuncture, and acupressure may also help in the treatment of many illnesses.

Avoid toxic exposures. It almost goes without saying, the best and easiest way to reduce the impact of toxins is to avoid exposure to them in the first place.

Eliminate alcohol and tobacco. No surprise here. Alcohol and tobacco poison the body and should be avoided. (For more information on stopping the alcohol or tobacco habit, see Chapter 11, "Overcoming Our Addictions," page 195.)

Sweat it out. Heat therapy—saunas, steam baths, tub soaks, and exercise—can help the body release both tension and toxins. Exercise is particularly beneficial, since it boosts metabolism and improves overall health. (For more information on exercise, see Chapter 8, "Working It Out," page 127.)

Quiet time. To rejuvenate your mind and body, you must rest and take time to center yourself. During detoxification, some people need more down time, but others feel more energized. In addition to getting plenty of sleep, consider performing relaxation exercises to balance the system and quiet the body and mind during detox.

TO EVERY SEASON

We need to detoxify our bodies regularly in keeping with the cycles of nature. We recommend that you detoxify your body when you feel congested (when we feel illness coming on) as well as during the change of seasons. (If the leaves change or the weather shifts, it's time for a detox.) We recommend a three- or seven-day fast with the change of seasons. These periods of detoxification give our bodies a chance to rest and prepare for the coming season. The more frequently you detox, the more you will be able to recognize and respond to your body's reminders for cleansing: There are times when each of us feels like eating lighter foods and eliminating more than we consume.

While short fasts can be started at any time, we recommended timing the fast so that it coincides with a weekend or other period when you can rest and allow your body to use its energy on healing and cleansing.

After a period of fasting or detoxification, you need to ease back into your regular diet, or better yet, into your new, healthier approach to eating. In general, we recommend that you take half the length of your cleansing to return to your regular diet. You don't want to shock your system with a full meal after cleansing. If you've been doing a water fast, begin by drinking fruit and vegetable juices. After reintroducing juices, move on to raw or cooked low-starch vegetables, such as spinach or other greens. As you expand your diet, be sure not to overeat. If you have trouble with a specific food, avoid it for a week or so, then try eating it again.

You might want to keep a diary during your fasting and detoxification, keeping notes on your physical and mental status as you work through the process. Your digestive organs, blood, and lymph system will be enhanced by the release of toxins and the opportunity for repair.

You will be surprised at the healing that can take place and the positive changes that you can make following a period of detoxification.

A SYSTEM-BY-SYSTEM DETOXIFICATION PLAN

Certain body systems require special consideration when it comes to detoxification. These include the liver, lymphatic system, kidneys, and lungs.

- **To detoxify the liver.** The liver stores toxic materials, then drains them into the small intestine through the bile. Every three or four months you should cleanse your liver by encouraging this drainage; the process can be encouraged by the use of certain nutritional supplements. Start with five or six drops of liquid phosphorus, available in health food stores. The phosphorus will help to thin the bile and make it flow more easily. Beets also encourage bile flow; add them to your detox juicing program during a liver cleanse. Dandelion leaves and artichokes also help cleanse the liver; add them to your regular diet. In addition, the use of psyllium seeds, gar gum, pectin, or oat bran can be helpful in binding toxins found in the digestive tract.

- **To detoxify the lymphatic system.** In order for the immune system to work its best, the lymph system periodically needs to be cleared of the toxins that it has stored. To do this, mix several tablespoons of castor oil and olive oil and apply this mixture directly over the skin to your underarms, neck, and groin area. Then take a bath in warm to moderately hot water to encourage the lymph flow. In addition, some massage therapists are trained in lymphatic drainage techniques; you may find it very invigorating to consult a specialist in this field. Goldenseal also helps increase blood flow to the spleen, which is part of the lymphatic system and assists in the detoxification process. One of the most important things you can do on a regular basis is to perform diaphragmatic breathing, which helps keep the lymph system flowing normally and helps mobilize the toxic material so that it can be moved out of your system.

- **To detoxify the kidneys.** The kidneys eliminate waste and toxins from the body; they need to be cleaned out every three or four months. Always be sure to drink plenty of filtered water (filter the water even if you drink from a well). Every few months use cranberry pills, available at health food stores, to help flush the kidneys.

- **To detoxify the lungs.** We are constantly inhaling dust and particulates from our environment. Our lungs catch these particles and then pass them upstream and out of the lungs using tiny little hairs. Proper breathing using the diaphragm can greatly encourage this process. Strenuous exercise also increases the depth of breathing and the release of toxins.

DO YOU HAVE A FOOD ALLERGY? USING AN ELIMINATION DIET

You may suspect that you have a food allergy. Every time you eat wheat, corn, or dairy foods, you experience diarrhea, bloating, and general misery. While your instinct may be correct, one of the easiest ways to find out for sure is to try an elimination diet.

The first step is to eliminate from the diet all of the most common allergenic foods, including wheat and other grains, milk and dairy products (including cheese), corn, yeast, refined sugars, processed foods, caffeine, alcohol, and foods containing preservatives, additives, and artificial colors. Do not eat these foods for four or five days, or long enough to clear all these foods from the digestive system.

Next, reintroduce the foods you have been avoiding one at a time. By keeping an accurate food and symptoms diary, you can identify the offending foods. You should test these foods again in three to six months. Most of the time, someone who is allergic to one food is allergic to many. It is often easiest to eliminate all possible allergens in the beginning of the test to get the most accurate results.

There are several variations to the elimination diet, including a water fast (water only for four days, then reintroduce the foods one at a time), dilute juice fast (juice only for four days, then reintroduce the foods one at a time), or the raw fruit and vegetable fast.

When introducing foods, add back the least allergenic first. Reintroduce foods in the following order: vegetables, fruits, melons, beans, yeasts, dairy products, and then grains. When adding dairy foods, reintroduce goat products first. If you don't have a reaction, add back plain yogurt, cheeses, and then milk. Repeat the process with cow's milk. Grains should be reintroduced gradually as well; test them in the following order: quinoa, amaranth, buckwheat, wild rice, brown rice, millet, barley, kamut, teff, oats, rye, corn, and finally wheat.

7
▼

Reshaping Your Body

Developing a Strategy for Weight Control

Anyone who has ever struggled with a weight problem knows that it isn't easy to be overweight. Society judges us; we judge ourselves. These negative feelings we hold on to about our bodies make it more difficult to lose weight. We want to disown the excess pounds; we want to amputate that part of us that makes us feel ashamed; we want to reject the image we have of ourselves. But this approach to weight loss does not work.

Before you can lose weight and keep it off, you must make peace with your body. You must accept yourself (whatever your size) and love your body (no matter how much it weighs). You must honor your fat before you can get rid of it. Your fat is a part of you; you are beautiful—that is the essence of unconditional love. Losing weight must be an expression of self-love, not a goal you seek to win the approval of other people.

Each time you eat you have an opportunity to love yourself. Once you learn to listen to what your body is telling you about what it needs and then to eat those foods that make your body feel its best, your metabolism will fall into balance and your weight will take care of itself. Any extra pounds will melt away without hunger or deprivation. You must learn to avoid foods that make you feel sluggish and impair your health, and replace them with healthful, whole foods that will nourish your body, mind, and spirit.

A MATTER OF HEALTH

Weight control is an important issue for African Americans. Nearly one out of every three of us is overweight. The older we get, the greater the problem: Forty percent of black men and more than 60 percent of black women are obese (more than 20 percent above their ideal weight) by middle age. These figures make African Americans on average the heaviest of all the major ethnic groups in the nation.

All those extra pounds take a toll on overall health, contributing to heart disease, diabetes, high blood pressure, gallstones, and some types of cancers, among other problems. In fact, experts estimate that obesity and weight problems contribute to more than 300,000 deaths a year. In addition, excess weight can cause problems with self-confidence and self-esteem, especially among women.

But there is hope: Lowering your weight can lower your risk of developing these life-threatening conditions. We have seen countless patients improve their health by getting their weight under control. By following a reasonable and well-balanced approach to weight loss, anyone can lose weight.

You may have tried to lose weight in the past and failed, but that does not matter. Today is a new beginning. You have another chance to love yourself. Do not dwell on past failures; focus on future successes. One patient spent most of her life dieting unsuccessfully. She was in her late thirties and weighed 265 pounds. We suggested she take a simple step and start walking—just one lap at the local high school to start with. She hesitated, but eventually started her walking program. She then restricted her fat and carbohydrate intake, and gradually increased her time on the track. Within a year, her weight had dropped to 160 pounds. She felt better about herself, which allowed her to meet new people. She met (at the track) the man she married; shortly after their marriage they participated in the Marine Corps Marathon. If you can visualize it, you can do it.

SIZING UP THE PROBLEM

We agree with the various experts who argue that too much body fat is hazardous to your health. You must be comfortable in your body; you must feel good about the way it fits. If you balance yourself energetically, you will lose weight (if your body needs to weigh less than it does) or gain weight (if your body needs to weigh more than it does).

Different people achieve this goal in different ways. You don't need to weigh yourself and establish a target weight in order to lose weight. In fact, one of the problems with measuring people is that if someone does not fall into the "desirable" part of the weight chart, they tend to judge themselves for being different. (As African Americans, we tend to judge ourselves harshly already; this just adds to our burden.) Rather than entering into competition with yourself, you can focus your energy on taking care of yourself and on eating healthful foods.

If you want to measure your body and monitor your weight loss, you can try calculating your "body mass index," or BMI. To determine your body mass index, multiply your weight (in pounds) by 705. Divide the result by your height (in inches). Now divide that result by your height again. For example, if you weigh 135 pounds and stand 5 feet, 7 inches tall (67 inches), your BMI would be:

135 (pounds) × 705 = 95,175
95,175 divided by 67 (inches) = 1,421
1,421 divided by 67 (inches) = 21 for a total BMI

Regardless of age, most healthy adults have a body mass index in the 20s. The risk of premature death rises as your body mass index rises above 25. Remember that the higher your weight or ratio climbs above the healthy range, the higher your risk of developing weight-related illnesses. If these measurements indicate that you have a long way to go to reach your goal, don't despair. Your journey must begin somewhere.

DR. WALKER: FORGET THE CHARTS

In order to lose weight, some people need to measure themselves and to have specific, measurable goals. I am not one of those people. I lost weight without using a scale. Ask yourself, "Has the bathroom scale helped me balance my weight and nourish my body by eating healthy foods?" If it has, keep using it; this method is working for you. But if it hasn't—if weighing yourself makes you judge yourself and if it undercuts your self-esteem—then toss out the scale and set yourself free. Instead of worrying about the scale, focus on your intention of self-loving. When you prepare your meals or sit down to eat, ask yourself, "Is this meal an expression of love and support for myself?" If you eat lovingly, you will achieve a healthy weight.

▲▲▲▲▲▲▲▲▲▲▲▲▲▲▲▲▲▲▲▲▲▲▲▲▲

▼▼▼▼▼▼▼▼▼▼▼▼▼▼▼▼▼▼▼▼▼▼▼▼▼

All Fat Is Not Created Equal

Pounds alone don't tell the whole story. One critical issue is where those pounds are located. Fat around your middle—in the abdomen and chest—is much more hazardous than fat around your hips, thighs, and buttocks. (As a rule, it's also much easier to lose.) If your fat gravitates toward your middle, you have an android or "apple" body type; if your fat tends to settle in your hips and lower body, you have a gynecoid or "pear" body type. Unfortunately, African Americans tend to be the more hazardous apple type when it comes to putting on extra weight.

It's more dangerous to be an apple than a pear because abdominal fat enters the bloodstream more easily than fat from the lower body, raising cholesterol levels and increasing the risk of cardiovascular disease. Excess weight around the waist is more likely to cause diabetes as well.

A quick look in the mirror can show you where you tend to pack on the pounds. Researchers have found that a waist measurement of more than 34 inches in women or 40 inches in men strongly correlates with other measures of obesity. If you want a more sophisticated measure, you can calculate your waist-to-hip ratio. To do this, measure your waist (in inches) at its narrowest point; then measure your hips at their widest point. Divide the waist measurement by the hip measurement. Women should have a ratio of less than 0.8; men, less than 1. A higher ratio indicates that you have too much abdominal fat and you should make an effort to lose weight, regardless of where your weight falls on the weight tables.

▲▲▲▲▲▲▲▲▲▲▲▲▲▲▲▲▲▲▲▲▲▲▲▲▲▲

UNDERSTANDING SYNDROME X

Being overweight affects the entire body, and it often triggers other serious health problems, including hypertension, elevated blood triglyceride levels, and diabetes or hypoglycemia (which often precedes diabetes). For reasons we do not completely understand, these health problems often occur in clusters. When a person experiences this constellation of medical conditions, we say that the patient has a condition known as "Syndrome X."

Regrettably, we see a lot of Syndrome X among our African American patients. In fact, we estimate that at least half of our African American patients who suffer from obesity also suffer from the other health problems associated with Syndrome X.

We suspect that patients with Syndrome X have developed an insulin imbalance due to the physical stress of carrying excess weight. In these patients, the pancreas may produce more insulin than the body needs, triggering hypertension. If someone has hypertension as a complication of an insulin imbalance and the insulin levels are brought under control through changes in diet and exercise patterns, then the blood pressure goes down and the person loses weight. In these cases, it looks like the weight reduction caused the blood pressure to go down, but there is evidence that the insulin level plays an important role independently. Both weight loss and insulin control are important, but we believe that the insulin level plays a more significant role than some experts think.

In terms of managing Syndrome X, weight reduction is essential. If a patient loses weight (in some cases just ten or fifteen pounds), many of the associated health problems will resolve themselves. However, since Syndrome X is a serious medical condition, the treatment of it should be done under the supervision of a medical professional.

▼▼▼▼▼▼▼▼▼▼▼▼▼▼▼▼▼▼▼▼▼▼▼▼

Do You Have Syndrome X?

Which of the following risk factors apply to you:

- Obese (more than 20 percent above your desirable weight, especially with "apple" weight distribution)

- Triglyceride levels 140 or over

- High blood pressure (over 140/90) or on blood pressure medication

- Hypoglycemic (your pancreas secretes too much insulin and there is an abnormally low level of glucose—sugar—in the blood)

- Diabetic (your pancreas secretes too little insulin and there is an abnormally high level of glucose—sugar—in the blood)

If you have four out of five of these risk factors, you have Syndrome X. If you have three of the five, you should consider yourself a borderline case and take steps to reduce your risks.

▲▲▲▲▲▲▲▲▲▲▲▲▲▲▲▲▲▲▲▲▲▲▲▲

SEVEN STEPS TO WEIGHT REDUCTION

Weight control is one of the most stubborn and frustrating health problems we work with. As anyone who has tried to lose a few pounds is painfully aware, it is much easier for most people to put on weight than it is for them to lose the unwanted pounds. But there is hope, even for the multitudes who complain, "I've tried every diet on the market and now I'm bigger than ever before." Even the most stubborn weight problem can be overcome if you're willing to follow a moderate and balanced approach to eating.

This is our seven-point prescription for weight loss:

1. **Avoid the seven deadly (food) sins.** After working with hundreds of overweight people, particularly women, we have found that African Americans tend to be sensitive to certain foods, especially wheat products, corn, dairy products, refined sugar, fried foods, white flour, and large amounts of red meat (more than four servings per week). Those patients who have had the greatest success with weight loss have done so primarily by reducing their consumption of these seven foods.

   One man in his thirties comes to mind: He tried every diet he could find but had trouble losing weight. He then learned about the hazards of these seven foods, took steps to avoid them, and dropped from 232 to 190 pounds in one year without "dieting" by monitoring his portions or going hungry.

2. **Stabilize your blood sugar levels.** If you are overweight, there is a good chance that your blood sugar levels are erratic and that your insulin levels are high. Fluctuations in your blood sugar can cause food cravings, weakness, and lightheadedness. Chromium is an essential part of glucose tolerance factor, a molecule in the body that regulates carbohydrate metabolism and enhances insulin function. To maintain stable blood sugar levels while losing weight, take a good daily multivitamin/mineral supplement and 200 micrograms of chromium twice a day.

3. **Discourage your body from storing excess calories as fat.** If you consume more calories than you use to perform your daily activities, your body will do one of two things with the excess calories: It will either store them as fat or store them as glycogen (energy) in the muscles. Garcinia (hydroxy citric acid) helps the body preferentially shunt calories into glycogen production rather than fat. Garcinia is available at health food stores; take one garcinia tablet twice a day before the two biggest meals of the day.

   When taking garcinia, many people feel energized. One patient who had been taking garcinia for several months ran out and she found she had significantly less energy during her workouts. When she mentioned her experience during an appointment, we explained that her change in energy reflected the change in the amount of glycogen in her muscles that could be used as fuel.

4. **Burn more fat.** Obviously, the key to weight loss is to "burn" fat or to shrink your fat cells. (Unfortunately, once you have a fat cell, it's with you for life; as you lose weight, your fat cells contract or grow smaller, but they don't disappear.) The best way to burn more fat is to participate in regular, vigorous exercise.

Exercise helps you lose weight because you burn calories both during and after your workout. Exercise increases your basal metabolic rate (the number of calories your body burns at rest), allowing your body to burn more calories even when you're sitting still. Studies have found that all it takes is thirty minutes of steady exercise to boost the metabolic rate for at least twelve hours. In addition, the muscle mass you build through exercise further revs your metabolic engine, since muscle burns more calories than fat, even when at rest. (A pound of muscle burns about forty-five calories a day, compared to a pound of fat, which burns fewer than two calories a day.) While low-calorie diets can lower your metabolism, exercise can stoke your metabolism, making it easier to lose weight.

Exercise also helps you keep the weight off after you lose it. Research comparing people who lost weight through diet and those who lost through exercise found that the exercisers found it easier to keep the pounds from coming back. One study found that among people who kept weight off for at least two years, 90 percent exercised regularly (at least thirty minutes three times a week), and of those who regained the weight, only 35 percent were regular exercisers. (For more information on exercise, see Chapter 8, "Working It Out," page 127.)

5. **Control your hunger.** If hunger pangs undermine your best efforts to eat a healthy diet, consider taking nutritional supplements to help control your hunger. Studies have demonstrated a link between weight loss and the use of papaya enzymes and pancreatic enzymes. Pancreatic enzymes increase the metabolic breakdown of fat and help take the load off the pancreas. Both types of enzyme

are available in health food stores; take one tablet of either enzyme three times a day with meals to control hunger, speed metabolism, and improve digestion.

Acupressure can also be effective in controlling appetite. To help curb the appetite, apply pressure or gently massage the tab of cartilage on the side of your face at the opening of the ear. Hold the point for several minutes when you feel hungry to see if it can help suppress your desire to eat.

6. **Satisfy your cravings—but not with food.** Many people overeat because their bodies are out of balance; food cravings often indicate that the body is deficient in certain nutrients. If your body is in balance, your metabolism will be more efficient and you will have fewer cravings. *Pica* is the word used to describe a food craving that is based in a mineral deficiency; in our diet, pica cravings often show up as a craving for sugar and salt. Eating sweetened and salted foods temporarily quenches the craving, but because the body is actually craving minerals (not sugar and salt), the craving quickly resurfaces. To minimize pica cravings, truly satisfy them by eating a balanced and wholesome diet and using nutritional supplements. (See Chapter 5 on page 85 for information on diet and Chapter 9 on page 149 for information on nutritional supplements.)

In addition, a lot of people crave sweets because their bodies don't make enough bile; this condition is especially common in people suffering from constipation. Olive oil helps improve bile flow, as does eating avocados. If you crave sugars, give these plant-based fats a chance to meet your dietary needs.

Sugar cravings can also be caused by hyperacidity, which often results from lack of exercise or eating too quickly, as well as by eating too much meat. Try eating same raw or lightly cooked vegetables or drinking a glass of tea with lemon. Try breathing deeply until the craving subsides. Take time to chew your food; the longer you chew grains, legumes, and vegetables, the sweeter they become. You might also try supplementing your diet with 500 to 1000 milligrams of the amino acid L-glutamine three times a day, which diminishes the body's desire for sweets and alcohol. (L-glutamine should be taken on an empty stomach.)

7. **Understand why you've gained weight.** To prevent future weight gain, you need to understand the psychological issues behind your relationship with food. Are you eating because you're bored? Sad? Angry? Or have you gained weight because you stopped exercising or started nibbling on snacks throughout the day?

It's important to analyze the issues that caused you to gain weight so that you can either change your environment or confront some of the more serious issues behind your weight problem. We encourage many of our patients to try Overeaters Anonymous or other support groups. Those who don't feel comfortable with a group situation may respond better to individual counseling. While many of our patients initially resist talking to a professional about their emotional issues surrounding food, in many cases people must change their psychological relationship with food in order to develop a more healthy physical relationship with it. Find professional support, if appropriate, to help you understand the psychological issues that caused you to gain weight in the first place.

A NEW WAY OF LIFE

If you need to lose weight, remember that weight loss should be slow and steady. If you try to drop more than a pound or two a week (either through diet or exercise), your body will switch into its fat-preservation mode and fight to keep you as plump as possible. Nature designed us that way: Whenever the human body loses too much weight too fast, hormones cause the metabolism to slow down and hunger pangs to kick in to prevent us from wasting away. Rather than go on a diet for weight loss (which has an implicit meaning that you are making food choices other than you would on a nondieting day), you need to focus on changing the way you eat and prepare food.

Alas, there are no magic formulas or weight-loss secrets that will make the task of losing weight quick and painless. The truth (as you already know) is that to lose weight—and keep it off—you must change the harmful habits and destructive thought patterns that made you gain weight in the first place. You must commit yourself to eating a well-balanced diet and getting regular exercise. That doesn't mean that you must swear off all of your favorite foods and become a martyr to the cause. In fact, drastic measures almost always fail. Instead, keep these tips in mind:

- **Say yes to fiber.** A high-fiber diet keeps the digestive system moving, it helps prevent certain types of cancer, and it fills you up so you'll be less tempted to snack on less healthy fare.

- **Add flavor to your life.** Don't add fat; instead use herbs, spices, and other seasonings. If low-fat foods taste bland and uninspired, punch them up with a trip to the spice rack.

- **Don't forget the most important meal of the day.** They're all important, but breakfast can be especially helpful in switching your body from the sleep mode into the high-energy mode. If you skip breakfast, you will drag through the morning (metabolically as well as in mood), and you will also be more likely to overeat later in the day.

- **Don't skip meals.** Breakfast isn't the only meal you should never skip. Skipping lunch or dinner can also cause your metabolic rate to drop. You will gain more weight if you eat a single 2,100-calorie meal each day than if you eat three 700-calorie meals. By spreading your calories throughout the day, you can actually eat up to 20 percent more calories without gaining weight.

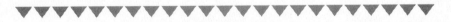

USE YOUR NOSE

Inhaling certain aromas can reduce your temptation to ingest food. In fact, researchers at Duke University have used apricot oil to help overweight patients at the university's weight-loss clinic control their eating. These experts already knew that many overweight people nibble and snack when nervous rather than when hungry. The researchers had the patients sniff the apricot oil while performing relaxation exercises. They learned to associate the fragrance with the state of relaxation. When they felt stressed out or anxious, the dieters could sniff from a vial of apricot oil rather than reach for an apricot pastry or another snack. More than half the compulsive eaters who tried the technique found that it worked.

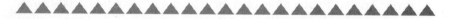

OUR HERITAGE OF HEALING

Nettle is an herb that has been used by the Caribbean people, as well as American Indians and many others, to help with weight reduction. Nettle is rich in mineral salts and vitamins, and may help alleviate "pica" cravings. If you want to give this remedy a try, prepare an infusion by steeping 2 to 3 tablespoons of nettle leaves in 1 cup of boiling water for 10 minutes. Drink 1 cup up to 3 times a day. You can also eat the whole plant by cooking it (perhaps with onion and other vegetables) in olive oil.

Working It Out

Exercise for Optimal Health

Danyell is typical of many African American women who struggle with their weight. When she came to the office, she weighed 212 pounds—far too much for her 5-foot, 8-inch frame—and she suffered from depression and high blood pressure. She walked out of the office with an "exercise prescription": Walk for twenty minutes three times a week. One month later, her outlook had improved, her blood sugar and triglyceride levels had dropped somewhat, her blood pressure was lower, and she had lost four pounds. While her weight loss may not have been dramatic, the improvement in her quality of life was astonishing; you can't just look to the bathroom scale for evidence of the healthful benefits of exercise.

Like Danyell, we all need regular exercise, but first we need to change the way we think about fitness. Too many African Americans consider regular exercise an act of self-denial, but, in truth, exercise is a way of honoring the self. As we've all heard time and again, exercise will strengthen the body as well as the spirit; it is an act of self-love.

At the same time, exercise can help connect you to your roots. When you exercise regularly, you will begin to feel a connectedness to all the things around you—the trees, the grass, the sky. You will be able to feel the pulse of your heartbeat in time with the pulse of the earth, energizing your body and rejuvenating your spirit. Our African ancestors appreciated the invigorating power of movement, and experienced the physical and spiritual rewards of exercise through tribal dance.

Still, as we've seen with so many patients, it is difficult to take the time and energy to nurture ourselves and our bodies, especially if we are bombarded with negative messages about our own self-worth. Allowing our bodies to grow soft and weak reinforces the message that we just aren't worth proper care. We can't tell you how often we have heard our patients tell us, "I'm too fat to exercise" or "I don't know what I'm doing and I don't want to look like a fool." These are nothing more than excuses and self-defeating messages; there is an exercise program for everyone, no matter what your size, age, or athletic abilities.

Some people believe that African Americans tend to be "natural" athletes, stronger and more in tune with their bodies than people of other races. While some of us do have gifts of strength, grace, and coordination, others of us do not. While we may be varied in our natural abilities, we do have one thing in common: Unless we take steps to preserve our physical fitness, over the years we will lose muscle mass and bone density while gaining body fat and excess pounds. Without regular exercise, even the most gifted athlete will lose aerobic capacity, muscle strength, and flexibility. Fortunately, it's never too late to get in shape—and stay in shape.

YOUR BODY WILL THANK YOU

The consequences of sitting still can be serious. Among African Americans, inadequate exercise is one of the major factors contributing to our overall poor health. The effects of too little time, too little money, and too few choices in convenient recreational activities have promoted the idea that exercise is a luxury that many cannot afford. On the contrary, exercise is a form of natural healing; it is a critical component of holistic health.

Exercise offers some of the best protection against many infirmities and illnesses. Some experts even suggest that some chronic complaints once thought to be major health problems may in fact be simple symptoms of disuse. You undoubtedly know you should exercise, but you may not fully appreciate how important exercise can be to your overall health. Consider the benefits:

- Exercise strengthens your immune system; after exercise, the number and aggressiveness of the white blood cells increase by 50 to

300 percent. It also increases the function of the body's natural killer cells, which are important in preventing cancer.

- Exercise reduces your risk of developing certain cancers, cardiovascular disease, colds and upper-respiratory-tract infections, diabetes (non-insulin-dependent), high blood pressure, osteoarthritis, osteoporosis, and stroke.

- Exercise relieves anxiety, constipation, depression, low-back pain, and stress, in addition to helping you sleep at night.

- Exercise helps to realign and clear the meridians, allowing for the free flow of energy throughout the body.

- Exercise helps to detoxify the body and eliminate metabolic waste through sweat and accelerated respiration.

- Exercise helps you maintain and improve flexibility, stamina, and muscle strength well into old age.

- Exercise improves your mood, mental alertness, short-term memory, and reaction time.

- Exercise can help you lose weight—and keep it off.

- Exercise can help people stop drinking and using drugs; the endorphin release during exercise can provide a "natural high" that can help an addict resist temptation.

- Exercise enhances sexual desire, performance, and satisfaction.

- Exercise helps make you look years younger than your chronological age.

- Exercise helps you live longer; some studies indicate that people who exercise regularly live as much as two years longer than their sedentary peers.

You don't have to spend hours in the gym working out as if you are Michael Jordan or Jackie Joyner-Kersee to enjoy the benefits of exercise. Recent studies have shown that as little as thirty minutes a day of light physical activity will reduce your risk of disease by lowering blood pressure and cholesterol. Yes, that's physical activity, not hard-core exercise. The time you spend strolling the neighborhood, walking the dog, climbing the stairs, and mowing the lawn counts toward your goal. Other studies have shown that you don't even have to do your thirty minutes of activity all at once as long as you total a half hour of total time during the day.

Of course, these studies looked at minimum levels of exercise. To enjoy all the benefits of exercise, you'll have to work harder and longer. But the point is that with a nominal level of exertion you can enjoy major lifesaving improvements in your overall health. In our experience, African Americans tend to respond to exercise and enjoy the benefits of exercise faster than people of other races. For example, we had a forty-five-year-old diabetic patient who had chronic back pain and fatigue. She was so physically limited at the time that she had trouble rolling over. Gradually she began increasing her exercise load; her confidence increased with her physical abilities. Her flexibility improved. Her pain eased and her blood sugar dropped to normal levels. She can now do multiple sit-ups—a task that was impossible before she started exercising regularly. She has lost weight, her back pain is gone, and she feels good about herself.

We can all learn something from this experience: Start where you are, take a small step, and enjoy the success of your accomplishment. Then move on, taking one small step at a time. Remember, it is not how much you do at first that matters. What matters is that you keep your promise to yourself. If you reach too far, you may set yourself up for failure and disappointment. Instead, start with something you know that you can do. Remember, the journey of a thousand miles must begin with a single step.

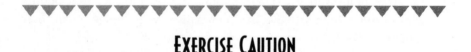

EXERCISE CAUTION

African Americans have a higher rate of sudden death during exercise than people of other races. That makes it particularly important that you check with your doctor before starting an exercise program if any of the following apply to you:

- You haven't had a medical checkup in more than two years.

- You're over thirty-five.

- You're more than twenty pounds overweight.

- You have high blood pressure.

- You have high cholesterol.

- You've had a heart attack, rapid heart palpitations, or chest pain after exercise.

- You're taking or have taken heart medication.

- Your doctor has told you that you have angina pectoris, fibrillation or tachycardia, an abnormal electrocardiogram (EKG), a heart murmur, rheumatic heart disease, or other heart problems.

- You smoke cigarettes.

- You have a blood relative who has died of a heart attack before age sixty.

- You have diabetes.

- You have asthma, emphysema, or any other lung condition.

- You get out of breath easily.

- You have arthritis or rheumatism.

- You lead a sedentary lifestyle.

▲▲▲▲▲▲▲▲▲▲▲▲▲▲▲▲▲▲▲▲▲▲▲▲▲▲▲

WORKING OUT A WORKOUT PLAN

"Fitness" means something different to boxer Riddick Bowe, Olympic ice skater Debi Thomas, basketball player Magic Johnson, and dancer Judith Jamison. While it might involve breaking a world record in the long jump for Carl Lewis, to someone out of shape it might mean being able to climb two flights of stairs or mowing the lawn without getting out of breath.

Although performance standards vary, we agree with those fitness experts who recognize four basic components of physical fitness:

- *Body composition:* The proportion of fat to bone and muscle.

- *Aerobic fitness or cardiorespiratory endurance:* The ability to do moderately strenuous activity over a period of time. It reflects how well your heart and lungs work to supply your body with oxygen during exercise.

- *Muscle strength and endurance:* The ability to exert maximum force is muscle strength. Lifting the heaviest weight you can in a single exertion is an example of muscular strength. Muscular endurance is the ability to repeat a movement many times or to hold a particular position for a prolonged period; for example, the work required to lift a weight twenty times or to hold it up for five minutes.

- *Flexibility:* The ability to move a joint through its full range of motion and elasticity of the muscle.

A well-rounded exercise program should develop each fitness component. But some people need more help in one area or another.

Body Composition

Body composition refers to your percentage of body fat, not your weight. You can't determine your exact body composition by consulting standard height-and-weight tables, but the tables can give you a rough indication of whether or not you're overweight.

More precise methods of determining body fat—such as underwater weighing and high-tech techniques using infrared light, sound waves, or electrical currents—require special equipment. But the low-tech, pinch-an-inch test can also help you determine your body composition. Locate a fold of skin and subcutaneous fat (the layer of fat beneath the skin) and pinch it between your thumb and forefinger. The back of the upper arm, the side of the lower chest, the back of the calf, and the abdomen are good places to test. After you pinch, measure the thickness of the flesh. If you can pinch more than one inch, your body has exceeded your optimal weight. For more information on weight loss, see Chapter 7, "Reshaping Your Body," page 115.

Aerobic Fitness

Let's look at our African ancestors. They were constantly active, walking, running, dancing, jumping. Physical activity was an integral part of their lives. You can bring this back to your life and allow your body's movement to connect you with your roots.

If you don't exercise regularly, you have almost certainly lost aerobic power—and you probably know it. Without exercise you will steadily lose aerobic conditioning throughout your thirties, forties, and fifties. By age sixty-five the average person's aerobic capacity has dropped by about 40 percent compared to the relatively fit days of young adulthood. Climbing a flight of stairs or walking through an airport concourse—activity that once caused little exertion—might now leave you winded and strained.

The term *aerobic* means "using oxygen." During aerobic exercise, your heart and lungs work harder than normal to provide your muscles with the oxygen they demand, and you must breathe heavily and steadily to meet your body's increased need for oxygen. During anaerobic exercise, your heart and lungs cannot meet your body's oxygen demands for longer than a short burst of activity, and you are left gasping and wheezing for breath (even if you're in good shape). Jogging around a track is aerobic exercise; sprinting to catch the bus is anaerobic exercise. No one—not even Carl Lewis—can do anaerobic exercise for more than a couple of minutes.

To improve your level of aerobic fitness and strengthen your heart and lungs, you need to perform some type of aerobic exercise, such as walking, jogging, bicycling, swimming, cross-country skiing, aerobic dancing, rope skipping, or even African dance (available at a growing number of recreation centers). These activities involve the rhythmic, repeated use of the major muscle groups. When done regularly—three times a week for at least twenty to thirty minutes—aerobic activities improve the efficiency of the heart, lungs, and muscles and increase their ability to do work and withstand stress.

Regular aerobic exercise helps lower your pulse rate both during exercise and at rest. As your heart grows larger and stronger, it pumps more blood with each beat, decreasing blood pressure. One study found that older people who had already suffered a heart attack reduced their risk of a second attack by 20 to 25 percent when they started to exercise. These heart-saving benefits show up after as little as six to ten weeks of regular aerobic exercise.

For maximum benefit you need to work hard enough—but not too hard. Your pulse rate, or the number of heartbeats per minute, is your body's speedometer: It tells you how fast you're going and if you need to speed up or slow things down to exercise in your optimal conditioning zone. Cardiovascular conditioning takes place when your heart beats at 70 to 85 percent of its maximum safe rate. Your maximum heart rate is approximately 220 minus your age. (See the table below.) You should take your pulse before starting to exercise, again after exercising for ten or fifteen minutes, and immediately after stopping.

Measure your heart rate at any place where you can feel your pulse. Two easy pulse points are the inside wrist and the carotid artery in the neck. Using a stopwatch, count your pulse for ten seconds, then multiply that number by six to get the number of beats per minute. During exercise a pulse that is under your target range indicates you should speed up or work harder, while one that is higher means you should slow down. Another simple test: You should be able to talk comfortably during exercise; if you can't carry on a conversation, you're working too hard.

Target Pulse Ranges

Age	Maximum Heart Rate	Target Range
25	195	137–166
30	190	133–162
35	185	130–157
40	180	126–153
45	175	122–140
50	170	119–145
55	165	115–140
60	160	112–136

65	155	109–132
70	150	105–128
75	145	102–123
80	140	98–119
85	135	95–115
90	130	91–110

If you're new to exercise, start slow. Try ten minutes of light to moderate exercise three times a week, and gradually extend your workout time to twenty or thirty minutes, then increase the intensity. If this is too much, start with what feels comfortable to you; the importance is that you begin. While our bodies need a certain duration of exercise for optimal health, you don't need to be a clock-watcher. The length of your workout is important only if you want it to be. Keep track of the time if that helps to motivate you, but don't worry about how many minutes you've exercised if monitoring times makes you feel unsuccessful. Listen to your body and over time you will develop a workout routine that is both physically challenging and spiritually fulfilling.

If you are over fifty, consider a low-impact activity; as we get older, the shock-absorbing fat pads in the feet thin out and the cushioning disks in the spine dry up, making high-intensity exercise more punishing on the joints. Remember that you can get a good workout using your arms; orchestra conductors tend to live into old age in part because they wave and swing their arms—often strenuously enough to work up a sweat—long enough to complete a concert.

Aim for workouts of moderate intensity—about 70 percent of your maximum heart rate. If you work at the higher end of the exercise benefit zone, you will experience a faster improvement in your athletic ability, but this extra effort won't markedly improve your health and it greatly increases your risk of injury. The death rates from cardiovascular disease, cancer, and diabetes are much lower in moderate exercisers than in nonexercisers. But the rates in heavy exercisers are only slightly lower than those of moderate exercisers. In addition, moderate exercise reduces stress, anxiety, and blood pressure as effectively as strenuous exercise does.

Be sure to warm up for five to ten minutes by doing light calisthenics before your aerobic workout. You might also go through the motions of the main workout at a slower pace as a warm-up.

Also remember to cool down. After your workout, walk slowly for three to five minutes, or until your heart rate returns to just ten or fifteen beats above the resting rate. (The less fit you are, the more time you'll need for a cooldown.) Stopping suddenly can cause the blood to pool in the legs, reducing blood pressure and possibly causing fainting or even a heart attack.

If one of your goals is weight loss, exercise is key. Try to work out frequently, slowly, and for a long period of time. Your body won't begin to pull from fat reserves until you're at least twenty minutes into your workout, so you should strive to design a regimen that involves five or six workouts a week, each lasting thirty to sixty minutes.

▼▼▼▼▼▼▼▼▼▼▼▼▼▼▼▼▼▼▼▼▼▼▼▼

GET WALKING

In Western cultures, we don't walk enough. Around the world, the main form of exercise is walking, and in Africa our people walk all the time. Walking, lifting, and carrying heavy things builds strength and cardiovascular endurance. You can enjoy the benefits of one of the most natural forms of exercise—walking—by making a commitment to a regular program of walking for exercise.

In addition to building cardiovascular strength, walking stimulates a critical acupressure point with every step. The point known as Kidney 1, which is one of the most powerful energy points, is located on the bottom of the foot, right in the middle of the ball of your foot. (To find the point, curl your toes; the indentation that forms in the ball of the foot is the correct acupressure point.) This critical energy point is stimulated every time you walk, with every step you take.

Just ten minutes of walking five times a week is extremely beneficial. Ideally, you want to work up to walking forty-five minutes five or six times a week, covering about three miles in the forty-five minutes. Start out with a short stroll, then gradually increase the length of time you walk and the distance you cover. You'll be surprised how quickly you make strides toward improving your health.

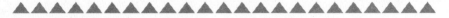

Muscle Strength

All too often African Americans confuse size and strength. We often speak to patients—especially men—who don't want to lose weight because they mistakenly believe that they are less likely to get pushed around if they are big. Strength and size are important in a society that tends to oppress the weak and small, but you don't have to be big to be strong—and you don't have to lose strength to lose weight.

Over the years, you will lose strength if you don't perform strength-training exercise. Many people assume that muscles atrophy over the years, but this doesn't have to be the case. You can keep your muscles strong and supple by performing strength-building exercises, such as weight lifting and isometric exercises.

Without strength training, you will lose muscle mass and strength: The average American loses 10 to 20 percent of muscle strength between the ages of twenty and fifty, and then another 25 to 30 percent between the ages of fifty and seventy. In addition, every decade from age forty on, the average person loses six pounds of muscle; this change in body composition from muscle to fat can change the shape of your body even if it doesn't change your weight on the scales because muscle is denser than fat.

Strength training helps stave off changes in body composition by raising the basal metabolic rate, or the number of calories the body burns at rest. The more muscle you have, the higher your metabolic rate, the more calories you burn, and the easier it is to fight flab. At age twenty, the average woman has 23 percent body fat; the average man, 18 percent. At thirty-five, those fat figures have jumped to 30 and 25 percent, respectively. And by age sixty, the average woman is 44 percent fat and the average man, 38 percent fat. That increase in fat corresponds to a decrease in muscle mass over the years.

To slow this shift from muscle to fat, you must do strength-building exercises, not just aerobic exercise. Studies have shown that people who maintain their aerobic fitness still lose muscle mass—about one pound of muscle every two years after age twenty—if they don't diversify their workouts to include strength training.

In addition to keeping you lean, strength training has other benefits:

- It makes it easier to perform simple tasks such as carrying groceries, opening jars, and climbing stairs.

- It decreases the risk of falls and injury.

- It strengthens the joints.

- It helps build bone mass and fight osteoporosis.

In fact, regular strength training can virtually stop the aging process when it comes to your muscles. For example, one study found that seventy-year-old men who had been strength training since middle age were just as strong, on average, as twenty-eight-year-old men who didn't strength train.

You're never too old to grow stronger. And the more out of shape you are, the greater your proportional gain will be. Frail octogenarians can easily double or triple their strength in just a couple of months. One study found that ninety-year-old nursing home residents increased their muscle strength by up to 180 percent in an eight-week exercise program. High-resistance exercise offers impressive benefits, even at age 101. When done properly, weight training has no great risk of injury or pain. And you can build as much muscle as—or more than—you had in your twenties.

We have had several patients who began exercising when they were older. One woman was quite overweight; she had chronic muscle aches, depression, and fatigue. She joined a walking class and her outlook on life changed as she began feeling better physically. Her muscle aches improved, her excess weight began to melt away, she rested well at night, and she reported that she felt more alert and energetic than she had in years. Once she started exercising her only regret was that she hadn't started working out years before.

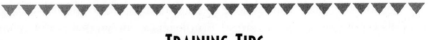

TRAINING TIPS

- Your training weight should be 70 to 80 percent of the maximum weight that you can lift. So if the heaviest weight you can lift in a certain maneuver is twenty-five pounds, your training weight for that exercise would be fifteen to twenty pounds. You should be able to lift that weight eight to twelve times. Once you can lift a weight twenty times, it's time to move up to a heavier weight.

This approach helps build "fast twitch" or "white" muscle fibers, which are responsible for strength. Muscles also contain "slow twitch" or "red" muscle fibers, which help with exercise endurance. To build these muscles, include weight sets that are lighter and perform more repetitions. As you approach fatigue, you will feel a burning sensation in the muscle as lactic acid builds in the muscle tissue. For this approach, do your initial weight set at 70 to 80 percent of your maximum, then mix in a set that is 40 to 60 percent of maximum (or lower). It is natural to feel achy a day or two after working a muscle group in this way. If your muscles feel painful longer than that, talk to a physical trainer or another health professional for advice.

- One set of each exercise is almost as effective as multiple sets in building muscle and boosting metabolism. However, to build muscle faster, follow a high-intensity strategy: After finishing the set, reduce the weight by ten pounds and perform as many extra repetitions as you can (usually three or four). This is called a drop set; you can keep lowering the weight with each set until you can lift only a few pounds. One two-month study found that people who followed the high-intensity strategy were able to lift twenty-five pounds more than before, compared to a fifteen-pound improvement among those who followed the one-set approach.

- Three workouts per week is the basic recommendation for building muscle. However, once you achieve the desired level of strength, you should be able to maintain that level with two strength-training sessions a week.

- To make muscles grow, work to the point of muscle failure, or to the point that you cannot perform another repetition of the exercise. Some experts believe the body needs to build up lactic acid inside the muscle cells to stimulate growth. Others believe that heavy weights tear the muscle apart and cause it to form new muscle fibers.

- Take it slow and easy. Each repetition of an exercise should take about six seconds—two seconds for the first half of the maneuver and four for the return to the original position.

- Use good form. Doing an exercise incorrectly can cause muscle damage and injury.

- Don't hold your breath. Holding your breath can cause a dangerous rise in blood pressure, then a sudden drop when you release your breath, possibly causing light-headedness or fainting. Inhale, then exhale during the exertion phase of the movement, and inhale during the release.

- Be wary of free weights. Start with weight-lifting machines or elastic exercise bands if your strength or balance have declined, since free weights can be dangerous if dropped.

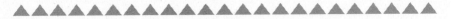

Flexibility

The dancers in the Alvin Ailey dance troupe epitomize physical conditioning. Their supple, toned bodies combine physical strength and aerobic conditioning, but it is the choreographed flexibility that makes the movements magic. While we may not all be able to control our bodies like dancers, we do need to spend some time working on flexibility.

Flexibility is a critical part of fitness but one that is often overlooked. Flexibility involves more than touching your toes; it involves maintaining the range of motion in your joints, which can allow you to perform your everyday activities without discomfort. It also makes you less prone to muscle strains, sprains, and tears. The only way to preserve your flexibility is to perform stretching exercises regularly.

Without regular stretching, the average adult's flexibility declines by 5 percent per decade. Over the years, that steady loss in flexibility can make it difficult to stoop over to pick up something dropped on the floor or to look behind you when driving.

As little as ten minutes of stretching every other day can help to prevent stiffness and loss of flexibility. Don't stretch "cold" muscles. Instead, stretch two or three minutes into your warm-up, just after you have broken a sweat. Stretch for two minutes before aerobic activities and ten minutes before abrupt, stop-and-go activities, such as tennis or basketball. You don't need to stretch before strength training, but you should afterward. Regardless of the type of exercise you perform, after your workout stretch two minutes for every ten minutes of your workout time. Stretching helps circulate your energy through your meridians both before and after exercise.

To build flexibility, bend or flex until you feel tension or slight discomfort—but not pain—and hold each stretch for twenty to sixty seconds. Do not hold your breath, and do not bounce or pulse, which can tear the connective tissue in the joints.

Building strength and increasing flexibility are not mutually exclusive. This myth has been perpetuated by people who build muscle and fail to work at stretching. Successful dancers and athletes know that they need to stretch before and after they train or perform—and so do you.

▼▼▼▼▼▼▼▼▼▼▼▼▼▼▼▼▼▼▼▼▼▼▼▼▼

Do You Need Special Nutritional Supplements for Exercise?

If you're in good shape, drink plenty of water, and eat a diet high in fruits and vegetables, you may not need to take any nutritional supplements other than your regular daily multiple vitamin/mineral supplement. However, if you're new to exercise, overweight, or don't eat as well as you should, we recommend that you take nutritional supplements. The general use of nutritional supplements is outlined in Chapter 9, "Enough Is Not Always Enough," page 149. In addition to the daily multiple vitamin/mineral supplement recommended for overall health, we suggest you add the following supplements until your body has adjusted to your exercise routine (at least three months):

Carnitine	500 milligrams twice a day
Chromium	200 micrograms a day
Coenzyme Q-10	30 milligrams three times a day
Magnesium	200 milligrams twice a day
Vitamin C	500 milligrams twice a day
Vitamin E	400 IU daily

WORK OUT, DRINK UP

You can't rely on your thirst to tell you when to drink during exercise. Instead, you should make a point to drink two 8-ounce glasses of water about two hours before exercise and another 8 ounces every twenty minutes or so during exercise. Then drink an additional cup or two a half hour or so after you finish your cooldown.

This water is necessary for your body to regulate temperature, carry nutrients, remove toxins and waste materials, maintain blood volume, and facilitate chemical reactions in your cells. You lose water throughout the day through urination, defecation, perspiration, and respiration (you release water vapor each time you exhale). When you're working out, you lose even more, depending on how hard you're working, as well as the weather and environment where you're exercising.

If you don't drink enough water, your body will let you know. You should check the color and quantity of your urine. If it's dark and scant, you're not drinking enough and your body is concentrating waste products in a relatively small amount of water. Urine should be pale yellow, and you should urinate at least four times a day.

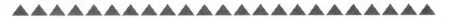

GET READY, GET SET, GET MOVING

No matter what your physical condition, it's never too late to start exercising, but don't expect to overcome decades of inactivity in a couple of weeks. It took a long time to get out of shape, and it will take some time to get back in shape, so be patient with yourself. You'll start to feel the physical and emotional benefits of exercise in a few weeks, and your fitness level will continue to improve over the next few months. Studies have shown that a year of regular exercise can return the body to a fitness level of ten years earlier.

Roughly two-thirds of all those who start an exercise program quit within six months. To get into shape, you will have to make a commitment to exercise regularly; sporadic exercise won't bring the rewards of fitness. Your body will adapt to the physical demands you place on it, and it will do so without injury or discomfort if you exercise sensibly. If you're not used to lifting anything heavier than a ten-pound bag of groceries, you'll find it difficult to lift a twenty-pound barbell. But if you gradually increase the demands on your body, your muscles will become stronger, and your heart and lungs will begin to work more efficiently.

You can challenge and strengthen your muscles in one of three ways: by increasing the intensity of exercise (the amount of weight you lift or the speed you run), the duration of exercise (the length of time you work out), or the frequency of exercise (the number of workouts per week). As a rule of thumb, limit the increase in intensity to no more than 10 percent per week to allow your body to adjust to your fitness program gradually.

You need to space your workouts for maximum benefits. If you perform aerobic exercise less than three times a week, you will not achieve adequate aerobic conditioning. However, if you work out five times or more, you run a much higher risk of injury and only a nominal increase in fitness. Perform your aerobic exercise every other day, with the strength-training sessions in between.

Once you start exercising, keep at it. Consistency counts. If you miss a few days of exercise, don't feel guilty and throw in the towel (literally). Instead, just get back to it, but don't try to make up for lost time by increasing the intensity of your workout. In fact, if you skip exercise for one week, cut back on the intensity of your workout and gradually build up again. You start to lose aerobic conditioning and strength if you sit it out for as little as one week.

TWO STRATEGIES FOR EXERCISE AND HEALTH

Regular exercise and physical activity should be your goal. We recommend that you strive to build time for regular exercise into your daily and weekly routine. Realistically, however, some people are not able (or willing) to make exercise a priority in their lives. For them, making a commitment to an active lifestyle may be the best they can do at the time.

As we mentioned earlier, you can enjoy many of the healthful benefits of exercise without spending hours in the gym. In fact, you can reduce your cholesterol and lower your blood pressure by spending as little as thirty minutes of activity every day. This "lite" exercise routine doesn't reward you with the same physical benefits a rigorous workout would, but it is enough to stave off the harmful effects of a sedentary lifestyle.

Here are two sample routines, which can meet the exercise needs of different individuals:

The Maximum Benefit Workout

To attain peak fitness (while still trying to minimize the time spent at the gym or working out), you need to strive to do aerobic training three times a week, strength training three times a week, and stretching for flexibility following every workout.

Monday	30 minutes aerobics
	10 minutes cooldown/stretching
Tuesday	30 minutes weight lifting
	10 minutes cooldown/stretching
Wednesday	30 minutes aerobics
	10 minutes cooldown/stretching
Thursday	30 minutes weight lifting
	10 minutes cooldown/stretching
Friday	30 minutes aerobics
	10 minutes cooldown/stretching

Saturday	30 minutes weight lifting
	10 minutes cooldown/stretching
Sunday	Rest

The Daily Living Workout

Several studies show that simply burning an extra 150 to 200 calories a day (or 1,000 to 1,500 extra calories a week) will provide some cardio-vascular benefits—and even help you lose weight and build muscle. To burn extra calories, you'll need to do at least thirty minutes of modest activity. (See the table on page 146 for a rough estimate of how much you'll burn doing some simple household tasks.)

Create a worksheet for yourself and keep a log of time spent in activity. For example:

Activity:	Mowing the lawn
Time spent:	20 minutes
Calories used:	110 (5.5 calories per minute × 20 minutes)

Activity:	Walking
Time spent:	15 minutes
Calories used:	68 (4.5 calories per minute × 15 minutes)

If you want to follow an active-lifestyle exercise plan, you will need to be conscientious about monitoring your activity level, at least in the beginning. Once you get a feel for the activity (and time) required to meet your goals, you can become less rigid about watching the clock.

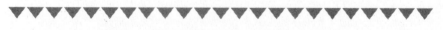

HOW MANY CALORIES ARE YOU USING?

The following list can give you a general idea of how many calories you burn doing certain daily activities. The estimates are for a 135-pound person. (The more you weigh, the more you burn.)

Activity	Calories burned per minute
Brisk walking	4.5
Mopping the floor	4.5
Washing the car	4.5
Weeding	4.5
Gardening (digging)	5
Roughhousing with kids	5
Mowing the lawn	5.5
Shoveling snow	6
Walking (fast)	6.5
Backpacking	7
Jogging	7
Walking upstairs	7
Running fast	13
Running upstairs	15

▲▲▲▲▲▲▲▲▲▲▲▲▲▲▲▲▲▲▲▲▲▲▲▲▲▲▲

▼▼▼▼▼▼▼▼▼▼▼▼▼▼▼▼▼▼▼▼▼▼▼▼▼

DR. SINGLETON AND THE POWER OF REST

The body needs rest. Not only is it okay to rest, but it is critical for your physical and mental health. You now have permission—in fact a prescription—to get one day of rest each week. It can be a Sabbath rest for religious or spiritual reasons, or just a "mental health day." But take it; it will help you maintain balance in your life.

When I was in medical school, I took a day of rest every week. I never studied on that day. People laughed and said there was no way I would make it through medical school. As things turned out, not only did I make it, but I graduated at the top of my class. I attribute a good portion of that success to the fact that I was better rested than my classmates.

The day of rest must be planned. If you leave it to chance to have time to play, it won't happen for most people. The same holds true of exercise. You don't need to do vigorous exercise seven days a week. Your body needs time to rest—and so does your mind.

▲▲▲▲▲▲▲▲▲▲▲▲▲▲▲▲▲▲▲▲▲▲▲▲▲▲▲▲▲

▼▼▼▼▼▼▼▼▼▼▼▼▼▼▼▼▼▼▼▼▼▼▼▼▼▼▼▼

Dr. Walker and the Power of Movement

I do not share Dr. Singleton's need for rest. I am a high-energy person, and if I slow down, I often find it hard to get going again.

I also graduated in the top 15 percent of my class in medical school, but I achieved my goal very differently. I studied all the time; that approach worked for me. Some people need to push themselves all the time; others need to rest to recover their energy before they push again. There is no single energetic approach that is right for everyone, so we encourage you to find an approach that works for you.

I may not devote an entire day to rest, but I do need to take "centering time" every day. During centering time you are still inside yourself, peaceful, and quiet in mind. Centering isn't vegging out in front of the television or snoozing on the couch; it is taking time to meditate, to work in the garden, to walk outside barefoot, to sit quietly with yourself. Centering allows you to sense the rhythm of the planet and to feel your place in the universe.

▲▲▲▲▲▲▲▲▲▲▲▲▲▲▲▲▲▲▲▲▲▲▲▲▲▲▲▲▲

▼▼▼▼▼▼▼▼▼▼▼▼▼▼▼▼▼▼▼▼▼▼▼▼▼▼▼▼

For More Information

- **Arthur Ashe Athletic Association, Inc.,** 355 Lexington Ave., 16th floor, New York, NY 10017, (212) 953-3100. The association provides support and resources for African American athletes.

- **Arthur Ashe Institute for Urban Health, Inc.,** 450 Clarkson Ave., Brooklyn, NY 11203, (718) 270-3191. The institute provides information on a variety of health-related topics, including exercise for African Americans.

- **The Black Women in Sports Foundation,** P.O. Box 2610, Philadelphia, PA 19130, (215) 763-6609. This nonprofit organization supports increased opportunities for African American women in sports.

▲▲▲▲▲▲▲▲▲▲▲▲▲▲▲▲▲▲▲▲▲▲▲▲▲▲▲▲▲▲

Enough Is Not Always Enough

Using Nutritional Supplements

Four years ago, a thirty-two-year-old African American intravenous drug user came to the office. She had been straight for several years, but she had already become infected with the AIDS virus. By the time we saw her, she was in the late stages of the disease. She had endured several opportunistic infections, her immune system was essentially wiped out, and she had tried a wide range of drug therapies. "If anything is going to work, it's going to have to be natural," she told us.

We put her on a diet of carrot and vegetable juice, organic foods, and supplements, including vitamin C, fish oil, evening primrose oil, antioxidants, and amino acids. This regimen combated the oxidative stress caused by the disease, and it allowed her body to control the inflammation and rebuild its defenses.

Within eight weeks, she gained weight, her energy improved, and her immune system grew stronger. After several months, she married and moved away from the area. We do not know what happened to her, but we were impressed that a woman who was expected to die in a matter of weeks experienced an unexpected rejuvenation and restoration of health when she offered her body nutritional support.

While this woman's health situation was extreme, almost everyone can benefit from taking nutritional supplements. Very few African Americans—in fact, very few Americans of any race—eat a well-balanced diet on an ongoing basis. Studies have found that more than half of all Americans have marginal nutrient deficiencies, and that figure jumps to an astounding 80 percent in some low-income communities.

Our poor diets contribute to our poor health. While problems related to severe deficiency are relatively rare, those associated with mild deficiency are quite common. For example, we don't see many patients with scurvy (caused by a lack of vitamin C), but we do see those who are deficient in vitamin C. Often these mild deficiencies cause vague symptoms, such as fatigue, lethargy, irritability, or difficulty concentrating.

Our African ancestors would not have needed to take nutritional supplements to meet their daily vitamin and mineral requirements because they ate a whole foods diet, which contained more nutrients than the typical modern American diet. The quality of the foods tended to be better because the soils were richer in minerals and free of pesticides and chemicals. But in the modern world, many of us don't eat as well as we should, and nutritional supplements provide some insurance that we get the nutrients we need.

Nutritional supplements help make up for some of the foods we aren't eating—and they help compensate for some of the foods we do eat that aren't so good for us. Studies have found that people who took a daily multiple vitamin/mineral supplement had stronger immune systems and suffered fewer infections than those who did not take the supplements. Supplements can also be used to treat disease once it has taken hold.

Some of our colleagues in the medical profession argue that most well-fed Americans get all the vitamins and minerals they need from their everyday diets. But our experience shows that our patients can improve their health and help correct illness and medical problems by using supplements. Recent research supports our position: Scientists have gathered exciting evidence that certain supplements may help control—or even reverse—many deadly diseases, including cancer, heart disease, and osteoporosis.

We have found that processed foods take a great toll on our African American patients' overall health. Consider the increase in the number of cases of asthma, especially among African American children. Recent studies have shown that high intakes of sugar and fat contribute to asthma, but why is this a problem now, when people have been eating a lot of sugar and fat for years?

The answer is frighteningly simple: The fats these African American children are eating consist of up to 40 percent trans-fatty acids, which have a negative effect on the mucous membranes, including the lining of the lungs. Children today consume more trans-fatty acids than ever before—and they suffer from more asthma than ever before. The trans-fatty acids, which can be found in margarine and processed so-called junk foods, also undermine the production of prostaglandins, increasing inflammatory problems and further contributing to the asthma problem. Changing the diet can help solve the problem, of course, but so can nutritional supplements. Nutritional supplements, including essential fatty acids, help to neutralize the trans-fatty acids and minimize their effect on the body.

A PRIMER ON NUTRITIONAL SUPPLEMENTS

Scientists have identified approximately forty different nutrients—including vitamins, essential minerals (needed in relatively large amounts), trace minerals (needed in relatively small amounts), and electrolytes—that are necessary for human health.

- **Vitamins** are organic substances that the body needs to regulate metabolism, assist in biochemical process, and prevent disease. Most vitamins are catalysts (or cofactors) in chemical reactions in the body. For example, vitamin B_5 (pantothenic acid) is a cofactor in a series of chemical reactions that burn carbohydrates. Vitamins are either fat- or water-soluble. As the name implies, fat-soluble vitamins dissolve in the fat; they can be stored by the body for long periods of time and can build up to toxic levels if taken in excess. Water-soluble vitamins cannot be stored and must be consumed every day or two; excess levels are eliminated in the urine.

- **Minerals** are basic elements; they cannot be manufactured or broken down by living systems. However, minerals do combine with vitamins, enzymes, and other substances as part of essential metabolic processes in the body. The mineral content of a plant varies from region to region and plant to plant due to variations in the mineral content of the soil.

Our Heritage of Healing

George Washington Carver was born a slave. He grew up during the Civil War in the foothills of the Ozark Mountains in Missouri, where he spent his early years working as a farmer and naturalist. He was one of the first people to realize that growing the same crop season after season caused a decline in crop production because it "mined" the minerals from the soil.

Carver experimented with several plots of land and learned that production could be increased by mixing old leaves from the forest, muck from the swamps, and manure from the barnyard in with the soil. He also found that rotating crops increased the nitrogen in the soil, increasing production. His contributions helped to improve the mineral content of the soil and to increase agricultural production in the South.

Unfortunately, our soils have once again been depleted by farming, irrigation, and acid rain. In fact, many of the fruits, vegetables, and grains available today are deficient in minerals because they are grown in fields with depleted topsoil. As a result, the foods we eat lack the nutrients we once obtained from them, making nutritional supplements more important than ever.

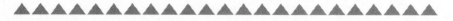

- **Electrolytes** are minerals that allow the transmission of electrical impulses in the body. They also help to balance the flow of water across the cell membranes, and they are essential to the maintenance of the water balance in the body.

- **Antioxidants** are a group of vitamins, minerals, and enzymes that help protect the body from the oxidative damage caused by free radicals. Many of our patients talk about the importance of antioxidants, but few of them really understand how antioxidants work in the body. Here's a basic explanation:

HOW ANTIOXIDANTS WORK THEIR MAGIC

Oxygen is essential to life. But at the wrong place and at the wrong time, oxygen can damage the cells, cause cancer, and contribute to aging through a process known as oxidation. As oxygen makes its way through the body, many of the molecules lose an electron, making them chemically unstable. These ions or free radicals are highly reactive; they strive for stability and ultimately "steal" an electron from another molecule, leaving a damaged molecule in their wake. This oxidative damage can cause changes to DNA, leading to cancer, as well as atherosclerosis, cataracts, arthritis, and many other health problems.

Antioxidants minimize the damage of free radicals by freely donating extra electrons, neutralizing the oxygen molecules before they hurt other cells in the body. Antioxidants include the well-known beta-carotene, vitamins A, C, and E, as well as the less famous quercetin, coenzyme Q-10, tocotriene, and lutein, among others. Antioxidants are found in many of the foods we eat as well as in nutritional supplements.

The link between antioxidants and reduced cancer risk is undeniable—though it is not fully understood. Literally hundreds of studies have showed that people who eat large amounts of fresh fruits and vegetables are much less likely to develop cancer than those who do not. What is not known is exactly how the antioxidants perform this task, or whether some other factor is at work. Fruits and vegetables contain antioxidants, as well as other compounds and nutrients that may also play a critical role in disease prevention either on their own or in combination. For this reason, if you want to hedge your bets against cancer and other diseases, eat plenty of fruits and vegetables. While there is conflicting data about the efficacy of antioxidant supplements, we recommend taking supplemental antioxidants as well.

- **Amino acids** are the chemical units or "building blocks" that make up proteins. In the body, protein makes up the muscles, ligaments, tendons, organs, glands, nails, and hair. Proteins are also included in enzymes, hormones, and genes. Amino acids may be joined in a number of different patterns to form more than fifty thousand distinct proteins and twenty thousand enzymes.

  The human liver produces about 80 percent of the amino acids our bodies need; the remaining 20 percent (the so-called essential amino acids) must be obtained from the diet and nutritional supplements. Amino acids are available in combination with various multivitamin formulas, as protein mixtures, in a wide variety of food supplements, and in a number of amino acid formulas. They can be purchased as capsules, tablets, and powders. Most amino acid supplements are derived from egg protein, yeast protein, or animal protein. The crystalline free-form amino acids are generally extracted from a variety of grain products.

THE DAILY DOZEN: KEY SUPPLEMENTS FOR ALMOST EVERYONE

While dozens of different nutritional supplements may be prescribed for specific conditions, we find that there are certain key supplements that prove useful for almost all of our patients. The following information can provide general recommendations on the use of nutritional supplements. We cannot tell you exactly which supplements to take and what dosage is appropriate for you without assessing your particular health needs. However, here's a rundown on the supplements we think belong in most medicine cabinets and our basic recommendations on using them:

Vitamin C

If there is one group of people especially in need of taking vitamin C, it's African Americans. The high level of stress, exposure to inner-city pollutants, frequency of cigarette smoking, and marginal diets increase the demand for vitamin C.

One-fourth of all Americans do not get even the minimum amount of vitamin C—60 milligrams—that cells need to perform basic biological functions. That figure is almost certainly higher among African Americans. In the body, vitamin C (ascorbic acid) serves a number of crucial functions. This antioxidant is required for tissue and collagen growth, wound healing, adrenal gland function, and healthy gums. It protects against the harmful effects of pollution, prevents cancer, and enhances immunity. It protects against blood clotting and bruising, reduces blood cholesterol levels and high blood pressure, and prevents atherosclerosis. It can be helpful in liver and colon cleansing as part of a detoxification program as well.

Consider the Evidence

- *CATARACTS*. Researchers at the U.S. Department of Agriculture's Human Nutrition Center at Tufts University suggest that cataracts may be caused by oxidative damage to the eyes. Studies have shown that people taking antioxidant supplements (including vitamin C) were less likely to develop cataracts than those not taking vitamins. A Canadian study found that cataract patients are only 30 percent as likely to have taken vitamin C supplements as those who remained cataract-free.

- *HEART DISEASE*. Researchers at the University of California analyzed the vitamin C intakes and death rates of more than eleven thousand men and women. The study showed a dramatic decline in death from heart disease among men with the highest vitamin C intake, especially among those who took a vitamin C supplement. Merely obtaining the RDA for vitamin C through food did not seem to offer any protection against heart disease.

- *GLUTATHIONE*. Glutathione is one of the most important antioxidants produced in the body. Low levels of this nutrient in the blood have been associated with cell damage and depressed immunity. Studies have shown that glutathione levels fluctuate with vitamin C intake.

People deprived of vitamin C had low levels of glutathione, but when those people were given a supplement of 500 milligrams of vitamin C, blood glutathione levels bounced back to normal.

* *CANCER.* More than 120 studies have consistently proven the cancer-fighting properties associated with vitamin C. Specifically, dietary intake of vitamin C appears to offer some protection against cancers of the lung, cervix, pancreas, mouth, throat, esophagus, colon, and stomach. There is also evidence that vitamin C may help to protect against breast cancer, especially in postmenopausal women.

* *LUNG DISEASE.* People who consume 300 milligrams or more of vitamin C a day were only 70 percent as likely to develop chronic bronchitis or asthma as those ingesting about 100 milligrams, according to a study of nine thousand adults by the U.S. Environmental Protection Agency.

* *SPERM COUNT.* Men who consume low levels of vitamin C are more likely to develop defective sperm than those consuming the recommended daily allowance of 60 milligrams. According to research done at the University of California at Berkeley, free radical damage to the genetic material DNA doubled in the sperm cells of men restricted to 5 milligrams of vitamin C daily (the amount in a teaspoon of lemon juice). When the men returned to a daily diet with either 60 or 250 milligrams of vitamin C, the DNA damage to sperm declined within a month.

Vitamin C is found in asparagus, avocados, beet greens, broccoli, Brussels sprouts, cantaloupe, cauliflower, collards, currants, grapefruit, kale, kiwifruit, lemons, mangoes, mustard greens, onions, oranges, papayas, parsley, green peas, sweet peppers, sweet potatoes, persimmons, pineapple, radishes, rose hips, snow peas, spinach, strawberries, Swiss chard, tomatoes, turnip greens, and watercress.

Some drugs—including aspirin, alcohol, analgesics, antidepressants, anticoagulants, oral contraceptives, and steroids—reduce the levels of vitamin C in the body. Diabetic and sulfa drugs may not be as effective when taken with large doses of vitamin C; large doses of vitamin C may cause false negative readings when testing for blood in the stool. Pregnant and breast-feeding women should use amounts of vitamin C no larger than 5000 milligrams a day, since infants may become accustomed to high levels of the vitamin and develop scurvy when supplementation is stopped.

Signs of deficiency include scurvy, bleeding gums, loose teeth, slow healing, dry and rough skin, loss of appetite. Signs of overdose include bladder and kidney stones, urinary tract irritation, and diarrhea.

R~x~ for Health

- Take 500 milligrams of vitamin C a day in divided doses if you are healthy. If you are sick, take up to 10 grams (10,000 milligrams) a day in divided doses. You need to divide the dose because you can saturate your body with, say, two grams, but in a few hours, you will need more. The body absorbs more vitamin C when it's sick than when it's not sick. For instance, most healthy people would develop diarrhea when taking 10 to 15 grams of vitamin C a day, but they can tolerate this much (or more) when sick with an acute viral illness.

- People who smoke need to take an additional 500 to 600 milligrams of vitamin C each day for every pack of cigarettes they smoke. We want you to quit smoking, but if you aren't ready to kick the habit quite yet, the least you can do to protect yourself is to take advantage of vitamin C's antioxidant protection.

CAUTION: If your body is deficient in the enzyme G6PD, you should not take supplemental vitamin C without consulting a doctor. If you have this condition, vitamin C can cause low blood sugar, dehydration, and diarrhea. People with this problem experience symptoms at an early age; if you think you might be G6PD deficient, talk to your doctor.

▼▼▼▼▼▼▼▼▼▼▼▼▼▼▼▼▼▼▼▼▼▼▼▼

DR. SINGLETON ON VITAMIN C AND KIDNEY STONES

Some doctors say that high doses of vitamin C can cause kidney stones. This is a subject I have researched extensively at the National Library of Medicine and let me say, for the record: There is no evidence to support the claim that vitamin C causes kidney stones in humans. Animal studies have shown that vitamin C at extraordinarily high doses can increase oxalate excretion, which forms kidney stones. For that reason, some people have avoided vitamin C supplements. The only people who need to worry about kidney stones are those taking more than 4 grams of vitamin C, and then only if they have a history of calcium oxalate kidney stones.

▲▲▲▲▲▲▲▲▲▲▲▲▲▲▲▲▲▲▲▲▲▲▲▲▲▲▲▲▲

Vitamin E

Vitamin E is another powerful antioxidant; it is especially important to African Americans because so many of us eat a diet high in fried foods and refined oils, which can cause free radical damage. However, vitamin E is not just for those who crave fried chicken and fatty foods.

Taking supplemental vitamin E can help to improve circulation, repair damaged tissue, and treat fibrocystic breasts and premenstrual syndrome, in addition to playing a role in the prevention of cancer and cardiovascular disease. It also promotes normal blood clotting, reduces scarring, lowers blood pressure, helps prevent cataracts, and helps slow the signs of aging.

Consider the Evidence

- *HEART DISEASE.* Several studies have shown a link between vitamin E supplements and a lowered risk of heart disease. In May 1993, *The New England Journal of Medicine* reported the results of an eight-year study involving more than 87,000 registered female nurses and a related study involving close to 40,000 male health care workers. The researchers found that those people who consumed daily vitamin E supplements (of 100 IU or more) for a minimum of two years had about a 40-percent (41 percent in women, 37 percent in men) lower risk of heart disease than those who consumed vitamin E through diet alone. (They also had a 29-percent lower risk of stroke and 13-percent reduction in overall death rates.)

In another study, sponsored by the American Heart Association, researchers found that long-term supplementation with 160 IU of vitamin E decreased the susceptibility of low-density lipoproteins (so-called bad cholesterol) to oxidation by 30 to 50 percent. Researchers suspect that when low-density lipoproteins oxidize they help to form atherosclerotic lesions in arteries.

- *CANCER.* A study sponsored by the National Cancer Institute suggests that people who take vitamin E supplements for at least six months cut their risk of developing oral cancers by half. Factors known to increase the risk of oral cancers, such as alcohol consumption and smoking, made no difference in the outcome.

  Other studies have found that vitamin E may help to prevent stomach cancer as well as other cancers of the gastrointestinal tract by inhibiting the conversion of nitrates, which are found in food, to nitrosamines, which are potentially carcinogenic, in the stomach.

  Vitamin E may help protect people from lung damage caused by chronic exposure to ozone in smog, as well as lung cancer among nonsmokers, according to two different research projects.

- *DIABETES.* A recent study done in Italy found that daily supplementation with 900 IU of vitamin E for four months helped people with type II diabetes better use insulin. Type II diabetes—also known as adult- or late-onset diabetes—accounts for 90 percent of all cases of diabetes. We had success using vitamin E (along with zinc and certain amino acids) to get diabetic patients off insulin. (See Chapter 13 on page 235 for more information.)

- *IMMUNE SYSTEM.* A study in *The American Journal of Clinical Nutrition* found that supplementation with high doses of vitamin E can enhance the immune system. In the study, thirty-two healthy older adults who were not taking any vitamin supplements or prescription medications were given either 800 IU of vitamin E daily for three days or a placebo. Those taking vitamin E showed a dramatic boost in immune function, while those taking the placebo did not show any change.

- *ARTHRITIS.* Several studies have shown that doses of up to 1200 IU of vitamin E can be as effective as a common anti-inflammatory drug at relieving pain, swelling, and morning stiffness caused by rheumatoid arthritis.

- *CATARACTS.* Studies have found that taking vitamin E supplements can lower the risk of developing cataracts by up to 56 percent, though vitamin C was found to be more powerful.

Vitamin E is found in cold-pressed vegetable oils, dark green leafy vegetables, legumes, nuts and seeds, and whole grains. Significant quantities are also found in brown rice, cornmeal, dry beans, eggs, liver, milk, oatmeal, organ meats, sweet potatoes, and wheat germ. However, it's virtually impossible to get enough vitamin E through foods without consuming large amounts of vitamin E oil.

The body needs zinc in order to maintain the proper levels of vitamin E in the blood. (See page 172 for information on zinc supplementation.) Vitamin E deficiency is most common in people with an impaired absorption of fat.

R$_x$ for Health

- Take 400 to 800 IU daily of vitamin E. People suffering from diabetes, rheumatic heart disease, or an overactive thyroid should not use vitamin E at high doses (above 200 IU). If a product label states the antioxidant content, check the label to make sure it contains at least 30 percent antioxidants; some inferior brands contain only 4 to 5 percent. Inferior brands also tend to be weaker, and they become rancid more rapidly. We tell our patients: Cheaper isn't better when it comes to vitamin E.

Selenium

Selenium is a vital antioxidant, especially when combined with vitamin E. This mineral was once considered toxic, but now it is considered essential for good health.

In the body, this trace element is used to form the antioxidant selenium-glutathione peroxidase. It is needed for pancreatic function, tissue elasticity, and red blood cell metabolism. It also appears to help stimulate antibody formation after vaccines.

Consider the Evidence

- *CANCER.* Studies have found a direct correlation between the death rate from cancer and selenium intake in food; in other words, people who eat the least amount of selenium have the highest rates of cancer. For example, in Japan (where the daily selenium intake is 500 micrograms) the cancer rate is more than five times lower than it is in countries where the selenium intake is 250 micrograms. Researchers have also found lower blood levels of selenium in cancer patients compared with healthy people. Other studies have demonstrated that selenium actually protects cell membranes from attack by free radicals.

- *HEART DISEASE.* Selenium helps prevent blood clots (which can cause both heart attack and stroke) and protects lipids in the blood from oxidation, a process that appears to contribute to the formation of atherosclerosis. Studies have linked a low selenium intake to a higher rate of both heart attack and stroke. For example, in Colorado Springs, Colorado, an area with one of the highest levels of selenium in the soil in the United States, the death rate due to heart disease is 67 percent below the national average.

Depending on the soil content, selenium can be found in meat and grains. It can also be found in Brazil nuts, brewer's yeast, broccoli, brown rice, chicken, dairy products, egg yolk, fish, garlic, molasses, onions, salmon, seafood, torula, tuna, vegetables, wheat germ, and whole grains.

R$_x$ *for Health*
- Take 200 micrograms of selenium daily.

Calcium/Magnesium

African Americans (as well as Asians) suffer more than people of other races from lactose intolerance, which makes us experience digestive problems when we consume milk and other dairy products. As a result, many of us don't consume enough calcium-rich dairy products to meet the recommended daily allowance of calcium. (Though dairy foods are high in calcium, they are also high in phosphorus, meaning the bioavailability of the calcium is low.) A good alternative source: green vegetables.

Calcium is vital in the formation of strong bones and teeth; it is also important in the maintenance of a regular heartbeat, transmission of nerve impulses, prevention of osteoporosis, and clotting of blood. It is essential for muscle growth and contractions, and may help lower blood pressure.

Calcium and magnesium must be taken together to work their best, with roughly twice the amount of magnesium as calcium. Magnesium protects the lining of the arteries from stress caused by sudden blood pressure changes, and it plays a role in the formation of bone and in carbohydrate and mineral metabolism.

Consider the Evidence

- *OSTEOPOROSIS.* Calcium can help reduce the bone loss associated with osteoporosis. French researchers gave sixteen hundred postmenopausal women 1200 milligrams of calcium and 800 IU of vitamin D daily for eighteen months; a second group was given a placebo. The results: a 43-percent reduction in hip fractures and a 2.7-percent increase in bone density on the hip among the vitamin-supplemented group; bone density fell 4.6 percent in the placebo group.

- *BLOOD PRESSURE.* Several studies have found that calcium supplements can help lower blood pressure. A thirteen-year California study of more than six thousand people found that those who consumed 1000 milligrams of calcium daily reduced their risk of developing hypertension by 20 percent. Another study of children found that those who ate the most calcium-rich foods had the lowest blood pressure.

- *CANCER.* Several studies have linked low intake of calcium and vitamin D with an increased risk of colon cancer. A nineteen-year study of more than fifteen hundred men in Chicago found that an intake of more than 375 milligrams of calcium daily (roughly the amount in one glass of milk) was associated with a 50-percent reduction in the rate of colon cancer and a calcium intake of over 1200 milligrams was associated with a 75-percent decrease in colon cancer. Researchers suspect that the calcium binds with fatty acids, preventing them from irritating the walls of the colon.

- *PREGNANCY-INDUCED HYPERTENSION.* Approximately one out of every ten pregnant women develops pregnancy-induced hypertension (PIH), a potentially life-threatening condition. In one study of 1,167 pregnant women, those who took 2000 milligrams of calcium a day had a 30-percent lower risk of PIH than those who did not take supplements.

- *LEAD.* Calcium protects the bones and teeth from lead by slowing or blocking the absorption of this toxic metal. In people with a calcium deficiency, the lead is absorbed by the body and deposited in the teeth and bones. This calcium-lead link may explain why there tend to be higher levels of lead in children who have a lot of dental cavities.

- *HEART DISEASE.* Epidemiological studies have found that people who live in areas with high levels of magnesium in the soil and water tend to have a lower rate of heart disease than the general population. Other studies have shown that people who have heart attacks have a lower-than-normal level of magnesium in their body tissues. As far back as the 1950s, animal studies have shown that high doses of magnesium can actually reverse atherosclerotic plaques. Other studies have shown that magnesium decreases blood pressure and improves the blood flow to the heart. In addition, studies have found that people who get intravenous magnesium after a heart attack have a significantly better survival rate than those who don't.

- *DIABETES.* Studies have shown that supplemental magnesium can improve glucose handling in people with insulin resistance. Other studies have shown that magnesium supplements can reduce blood pressure and lower the risk of complications in patients who already have diabetes.

Sources of calcium include kale, parsley, salmon (with bones), sardines, and seafood. In addition, calcium is found in almonds, asparagus, blackstrap molasses, brewer's yeast, broccoli, buttermilk, cabbage, carob, collard greens, cow's milk, dandelion greens, figs, goat's milk, kelp, mustard greens, oats, prunes, sesame seeds, spinach, tofu, turnip greens, whey, and yogurt. (Most calcium supplements come from inorganic sources and have about a 3-percent absorption rate; calcium from plants, on the other hand, has an absorption rate of 30 to 50 percent.)

Magnesium is found in most foods, especially dairy products, fish, meat, and seafood. Other rich food sources include apples, apricots, avocados, bananas, blackstrap molasses, brewer's yeast, brown rice, figs, garlic, kelp, lima beans, millet, nuts, peaches, black-eyed peas, salmon, sesame seeds, shrimp, tofu, green leafy vegetables, wheat, and whole grains.

Calcium supplements should not be taken by people suffering from kidney stones or kidney disease or by those taking calcium channel blockers for the heart. Calcium taken with iron reduces the effect of both minerals, so take them at different times of day.

Signs of calcium deficiency include muscle cramps, nervousness, heart palpitations, brittle nails, eczema, hypertension, aching joints, increased cholesterol levels, rheumatoid arthritis, tooth decay, insomnia, rickets, and numbness in the arms or legs. Calcium deficiency can also cause rickets in children and osteoporosis in adults. Signs of calcium overdose include drowsiness, calcium deposits, and impaired absorption of iron and other minerals.

Use of alcohol or diuretics (water pills), or chronic diarrhea, increases the body's need for magnesium. Large amounts of fats, cod liver oil, calcium, vitamin D, and protein decrease magnesium absorption. Symptoms of magnesium deficiency include muscle tremors, leg cramps, weakness, irregular heartbeat, constipation, and chronic low potassium levels. Signs of magnesium overdose include upset in calcium-magnesium ratio, resulting in impaired nervous system function. We have had several patients with heart palpitations whose condition has resolved after taking magnesium supplements; it can also be helpful in the treatment of asthma.

R_x for Health

- Most people should take 1000 milligrams of calcium and 2000 milligrams of magnesium daily. Menopausal women should take 1500 milligrams of calcium and 3000 milligrams of magnesium daily. These minerals are more easily absorbed by the body when taken in divided doses throughout the day. Calcium in the form of calcium citrate is more readily absorbed by the body than calcium in other forms.

▼▼▼▼▼▼▼▼▼▼▼▼▼▼▼▼▼▼▼▼▼▼▼▼

The Dilution Solution

Do you wonder whether the calcium pills you swallow are sufficiently broken down in your stomach? To find out, try this simple test. Place a calcium pill in a glass of warm water and shake. If the pill does not break down within twenty-four hours, change to another brand or form of calcium and repeat the experiment. Keep in mind, however, that the best and most bioavailable forms of calcium (and magnesium) are found in plants, not pills.

▲▲▲▲▲▲▲▲▲▲▲▲▲▲▲▲▲▲▲▲▲▲▲▲

▼▼▼▼▼▼▼▼▼▼▼▼▼▼▼▼▼▼▼▼▼▼▼▼

Dr. Walker on Calcium Supplements

I have significant concerns regarding the long-term use of inorganic calcium supplements. Calcium works as a charged particle or ion. In this ionized form, it can enter cells and be used. When calcium comes from nonplant, nonanimal sources, it is not easily used by the body. I am one of a growing number of practitioners who believe that inorganic calcium can "clump up" in the system, contributing to health problems such as kidney stones and gallstones, as well as the formation of calcium deposits in the arteries and tissues.

I recommend using plant-based calcium and magnesium; an excellent source is green barley, also known as green magma. It is available in health food stores; follow package directions for dosage information.

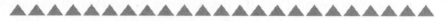

Vitamin A and Beta-carotene

Vitamin A and beta-carotene are closely related nutrients. Preformed vitamin A (called retinol) is found in animal tissues. Beta-carotene is a pigment found in plant foods (especially yellow and orange vegetables and fruits). Because it can be converted to vitamin A in the intestinal tract or liver, beta-carotene is sometimes called provitamin A. Vitamin A can be toxic at high doses; beta-carotene is not considered toxic (though it can turn your skin somewhat orange at very large doses).

Vitamin A deficiency is a common cause of eye disease worldwide, and some of the people who come to the United States from Africa suffer from compromised vision due to vitamin deficiencies. Fortunately, most of the time these problems can be reversed with nutritional supplements.

Vitamin A and beta-carotene prevent night blindness and other eye problems as well as some skin disorders such as acne. They are antioxidants, and so they enhance immunity, reduce the signs of aging, and protect the body from free radical damage. They also heal gastrointestinal ulcers, assist in the maintenance and repair of epithelial tissue, and help with the formation of bones and teeth.

Consider the Evidence

- *CANCER.* A number of studies conducted worldwide have linked low beta-carotene intake and low blood levels of beta-carotene with an increased risk of many different forms of cancer, including cancer of the breast, cervix, lung, stomach, colon and rectum, bladder, mouth, and esophagus. A Johns Hopkins University study found that people with low blood levels of beta-carotene were four times more likely to develop lung cancer due to smoking. On the other hand, a 1994 Finnish study found that large doses of beta-carotene failed to prevent lung cancer in smokers, but this study looked at beta-carotene taken in pill form rather than as whole foods.

• *HEART DISEASE.* Population studies have found that people with a high intake of beta-carotene have a lower rate of heart disease than those who don't. For example, ongoing research in the Nurses' Health Study shows that by eating even one serving of fruits or vegetables daily, you can reduce your risk of heart attack and stroke. Women in the study who took between 15 and 20 milligrams of beta-carotene daily had a 22-percent reduced risk of heart attack and a 37-percent reduced risk of stroke.

Taking supplements can help, too. A Harvard study showed that male physicians who took a 50-milligram supplement of beta-carotene every other day for six years had only half as many fatal heart attacks and strokes as doctors who took a placebo. The protective effect showed up only after taking the supplements for two years, suggesting that beta-carotene slows the buildup of plaque in the arteries.

• *IMMUNITY.* Beta-carotene supplements support the body's immune system. A study at the University of Arizona found that those people who took 30 to 60 milligrams of beta-carotene daily for two months had more natural killer cells, T helper cells, and activated lymphocytes than people taking a placebo. These immune cells help protect the body from cancer and viral and bacterial infections. Another study found that Harvard physicians taking 50 milligrams of beta-carotene every other day had a significant rise in the number of immune-boosting natural killer cells in their blood, which are particularly important in fighting off cancer.

Vitamin A or beta-carotene can be found in fish liver oils, animal livers, and green and yellow fruits and vegetables. Other foods that contain vitamin A include alfalfa, apricots, asparagus, beets, broccoli, cantaloupe, carrots, Swiss chard, dandelion greens, fish liver oil and liver, garlic, kale, mustard, papayas, parsley, peaches, red peppers, sweet potatoes, spinach, pumpkin and yellow squash, turnip greens, and watercress.

Vitamin A and beta-carotene should be taken with caution in pill form or as cod liver oil by people with liver disease. Pregnant women should avoid consuming more than 10,000 IU, since studies have found that higher amounts in the first trimester can cause serious birth defects. Antibiotics, laxatives, and some cholesterol-lowering drugs can interfere with vitamin A absorption. Diabetics and people with hypothyroidism should consider avoiding beta-carotene because their bodies may not be able to convert it into vitamin A.

Signs of vitamin A deficiency include night blindness, retarded growth, impaired resistance to disease, infection, rough skin, and dry eyes. Signs of vitamin A overdose include headaches, blurred vision, skin rash, extreme fatigue, diarrhea, nausea, loss of appetite, hair loss, menstrual irregularities, liver damage, and dizziness. No vitamin overdose can occur with beta-carotene, although the skin may turn slightly yellow-orange in color.

R𝗑 for Health

- Take 5000 IU of vitamin A or 10,000 IU of beta-carotene. (The 10,000 IU of beta-carotene will convert to about 5000 IU of vitamin A in the body.) In addition, be sure to eat a diet high in beta-carotene–rich orange-yellow vegetables and fruits.

B Complex Vitamins

The B vitamins help to maintain healthy nerves, skin, eyes, hair, liver, and mouth, as well as muscle tone in the gastrointestinal tract. B-complex vitamins are coenzymes involved in energy production and may be useful for treating depression or anxiety. The B vitamins should always be taken together, but up to two to three times more of one B vitamin than another can be taken for a particular disorder. Although the B vitamins are a team, we tend to use three B vitamins more than the others—B_5, B_6, and B_{12}.

Vitamin B_5 (pantothenic acid) is known as the antistress vitamin. It plays a role in the production of the adrenal hormones and the formation of antibodies. It aids in the body's use of vitamins and helps to convert fats, carbohydrates, and proteins into energy. Vitamin B_5 is required by all cells in the body and is concentrated in the organs. It is also needed for normal functions of the gastrointestinal tract and may be helpful in treating depression and anxiety.

Vitamin B_6 (pyridoxine) is involved in more bodily functions than any other single nutrient. It affects both physical and mental health. It is beneficial if you suffer from water retention. It is necessary in the production of hydrochloric acid and the absorption of fats and protein. Vitamin B_6 also aids in maintaining sodium and potassium balance, and promotes red blood cell formation. It is required by the nervous system, and is needed for normal brain function and for the synthesis of RNA and DNA, which contain the genetic instructions for the reproduction of all cells and for normal cellular growth. It activates many enzymes and aids in B_{12} absorption, immune system function, and antibody production.

Vitamin B_{12} (cyanocobalamin) is needed to prevent anemia. It aids in cell formation and cellular longevity. This vitamin is also required for proper digestion, absorption of foods, protein synthesis, and metabolism of carbohydrates and fats. In addition, vitamin B_{12} prevents nerve damage, maintains fertility, and promotes normal growth and development.

Consider the Evidence

- *ARTHRITIS.* One study of 189 people with arthritis found that those given a B complex supplement (including 100 milligrams of vitamin B_1, 100 milligrams of B_6, and 0.5 milligram of B_{12}) experienced significantly less pain than those people in the control group.

- *HEART DISEASE.* Vitamin B_6 helps to inhibit the formation of homocysteine, which attacks the heart muscle and allows the deposition of cholesterol around the heart arteries.

- *KIDNEY STONES.* Vitamin B_6 helps prevent kidney stones and acts as a mild diuretic.

- *PREMENSTRUAL SYNDROME.* Vitamin B_6 reduces the symptoms of premenstrual syndrome.

- *CARPAL TUNNEL SYNDROME.* Carpal tunnel syndrome has been linked to vitamin B_6 deficiency, and supplemental B_6 can be helpful in treating the condition.

Vitamin B_5 is found in beans, beef, eggs, saltwater fish, pork, fruits, fresh vegetables, and whole wheat. It is also produced by intestinal bacteria.

Even though B_5 is present in a lot of foods, the refining of foods will decrease the amount of B_5, so many people are getting less than they need. People who eat a diet high in refined sugars and flours and deficient in whole grains, fruits, and vegetables are probably not getting enough B vitamins. Signs of deficiency include fatigue, numbness, and mood swings. Signs of overdose include a thiamine deficiency.

All foods contain small amounts of vitamin B_6. However, the following foods have high amounts: brewer's yeast, carrots, chicken, eggs, fish, meat, peas, spinach, sunflower seeds, walnuts, and wheat germ. Other good sources include avocado, bananas, beans, blackstrap molasses, brown rice and other whole grains, cabbage, cantaloupe, and potatoes.

Antidepressants, estrogen, and oral contraceptives may increase the need for vitamin B_6 in the body. Signs of deficiency include confusion, convulsions, depression, irritability, insomnia, itchy skin, reduced resistance to infection, and sores in the mouth.

The largest amounts of B_{12} are found in blue cheese, cheese, clams, eggs, herring, kidney, liver, mackerel, milk, pork, seafood, tofu, and yogurt. B_{12} is not found in vegetables; it is available only from animal sources.

Anti-gout medications, anticoagulant drugs, and potassium supplements may block the absorption of B_{12} in the digestive tract. Vegetarians need this supplement because it is found mostly in animal sources. A vitamin B_{12} deficiency can be caused by malabsorption, which is most common in the elderly and in those with digestive disorders. Symptoms of deficiency include abnormal gait, memory loss, hallucinations, eye disorders, anemia, and digestive disorders.

R_x *for Health*

- Take 10 milligrams of vitamin B_5, 50 milligrams of vitamin B_6, and 10 micrograms of vitamin B_{12} daily. You might also consider a B-complex formula that includes a combination of B vitamins.

Folate or Folic Acid

Folic acid is needed for energy production and the formation of red blood cells. It is necessary for DNA synthesis, making it critical for healthy cell division and replication. Folic acid helps with fetal development; it is a crucial vitamin for pregnant women. This nutrient may also help in the treatment of depression and anxiety. Folic acid works best when combined with vitamin B_{12}.

Consider the Evidence

- *HEART DISEASE.* Folic acid helps prevent heart disease by helping to maintain normal levels of homocysteine, an amino acid found in the body. Researchers at Harvard Medical School found that men with even slightly elevated levels of homocysteine were three times more likely to have a heart attack than men with the lowest levels. Based on the study, when most men are given a folic acid supplement, homocysteine levels drop back to normal.

- *CANCER.* Researchers at Brigham and Women's Hospital in Boston have linked a diet low in folic acid to a change in DNA that may allow cancer-causing genes to take hold. In the study of 26,000 men and women, those with the lowest intake of folic acid had the highest level of precancerous tumors of the colon or rectum. Low levels of folic acid have also been linked to cervical cancer.

Good food sources of folic acid include avocados, barley, beans, beef, bran, brewer's yeast, brown rice, cheese, chicken, dates, green leafy vegetables, lamb, legumes, lentils, liver, milk, oranges, organ meats, split peas, port, root vegetables, salmon, tuna, wheat germ, whole wheat, and yeast.

Oral contraceptives may increase the need for folic acid. High doses for extended periods should be avoided by anyone with a hormone-related cancer or convulsive disorder. Inadequate intake during pregnancy increases the risk of spina bifida and other birth defects. A sore, red tongue is one of the most common signs of folic acid deficiency.

R$_x$ *for Health*

- Take 400 micrograms of folic acid daily.

Zinc

Zinc is a mineral important in prostate gland function and the growth of the reproductive organs. It is required for protein synthesis and collagen formation and promotes a healthy immune system and the efficient healing of wounds. Zinc also allows acuity of taste and smell and protects the liver from chemical damage. Zinc is also necessary for the red blood cells to move carbon dioxide away from the tissues; it is involved in the metabolism of carbohydrates and vitamins. Liquid zinc and zinc picolinate are the forms most easily absorbed by the body.

Consider the Evidence

- *IMMUNE SYSTEM.* Several studies have found a deficiency of zinc in older people with compromised immune systems. One study found that zinc supplements (220 milligrams twice daily for one month) increased the level of infection-fighting T cells in people over age seventy. In general, however, researchers have found that daily zinc supplements of more than 100 milligrams can depress the immune system while dosages under 100 milligrams can enhance the immune response.

- *COMMON COLD.* Zinc is a potent cold fighter. Zinc lozenges have been found to reduce the duration of colds by more than 40 percent (from an average of nine days to five days); zinc also reduces the intensity of cold symptoms. In the study, the participants battling a cold sucked on two zinc gluconate lozenges every two hours, up to eight per day. (NOTE: Zinc lozenges should not be taken on an empty stomach because they can cause nausea.)

- *INFERTILITY.* A number of studies have linked zinc deficiency to infertility and sperm problems in men. A study at the University of Rochester Medical Center in New York found significant improvement in the semen quality of men who took a daily zinc supplement for between two months and two years.

Zinc is found in fish, legumes, meats, milk, oysters, poultry, seafood, and whole grains. Significant quantities of zinc are found in brewer's yeast, egg yolk, lamb chops, lima beans, liver, mushrooms, pecans, pumpkin seeds, sardines, seeds, soy lecithin, soybeans, and sunflower seeds.

Zinc levels may be lowered by diarrhea, kidney disease, cirrhosis of the liver, and diabetes. The proper copper and zinc balance should be maintained. Consumption of hard water can upset zinc levels, as can the use of birth control pills.

R$_x$ for Health
- Take 25 to 50 milligrams of zinc daily. If you take more than 50 milligrams of zinc, you should also take supplemental copper at a ratio of 20:1. (Some products combine zinc and copper in the appropriate ratios.)

Chromium

Most African Americans don't get enough chromium from the foods they eat. According to a study published in *The American Journal of Clinical Nutrition,* more than 90 percent of American diets fail to meet the recommended minimum intake of 50 micrograms of chromium daily. And those people who eat a diet high in sugar and refined foods need chromium even more, but their bodies take in even less.

In the body, chromium (also known as glucose tolerance factor, or GTF) is essential for maintaining stable blood sugar levels. People who eat a lot of sugary foods need extra chromium, but the sugar actually destroys what little dietary chromium they take in. This imbalance can lead to blood sugar problems, such as hypoglycemia and diabetes. Both table sugar and high-fructose corn syrup (as found in soft drinks and other processed foods) can wash chromium right out of the body.

In addition, chromium is vital in the synthesis of cholesterol, fats, and protein. Low blood plasma levels of chromium are an indication of coronary artery disease.

Consider the Evidence

- *DIABETES.* Insulin helps the body metabolize glucose (or blood sugar) into a form that can be used by the cells for energy. Animal studies have shown that chromium helps regulate the release of insulin by acting on insulin-producing cells, or beta cells. Beta cells in the pancreas manufacture and store insulin until a rising blood sugar level signals them to release it. Animal studies show that chromium directly stimulates the production of insulin as the body needs it.

- *HEART DISEASE.* Several studies have shown that chromium can cut blood serum cholesterol levels and triglycerides, helping to prevent heart disease. One study found that when people with elevated cholesterol levels (220 to 320 milligrams per deciliter) were given either 200 micrograms of chromium picolinate supplement or a placebo, those given chromium experienced an average 7-percent drop in cholesterol after six weeks.

- *CHOLESTEROL.* A number of studies show that chromium helps to lower "bad" (low-density lipoprotein, LDL) cholesterol and raise "good" (high-density lipoprotein, HDL) cholesterol. One study found that giving people 200 micrograms of chromium daily boosted HDL levels by 11 percent. Another eight-week study found that men who received 200 micrograms of niacin-bound chromium showed an average drop of 14 percent in total cholesterol.

In their natural state, all carbohydrates have chromium. But any time the carbohydrates are refined, chromium is lost. For example, sugarcane and sugar beets are packed with chromium, but refined white sugar is not. In this case, the chromium (and most of the other nutrients) remain in the nutrient-rich molasses, which is a by-product of refining sugar.

Chromium is found in beer, brewer's yeast, brown rice, cheese, meat, and whole grains. It may also be found in dried beans, corn and corn oil, dairy products, calves' liver, mushrooms, and potatoes. It's almost impossible to get enough chromium from food. You have to eat at least 3000 calories a day to get about 50 micrograms—and even more to get the recommended 200 micrograms. Instead of overeating, take a chromium supplement.

Signs of chromium deficiency include infertility, cloudy corneas, and atherosclerosis.

R$_x$ for Health
- Take 200 micrograms of chromium daily.

Essential Fatty Acids

In the 1970s, some observant scientists noticed that Eskimos eat a lot of fat but have an exceptionally low rate of heart disease and cancer. Further study found that the fat in the Eskimo diet was primarily in the form of omega-3 fatty acids, which are found in fatty fish. Over the years, a number of other studies have supported the observation that omega-3 fatty acids in fact do help prevent heart disease and cancer.

Omega-3 is one of several essential fatty acids; these acids cannot be made by the body and must be supplied through the diet. Essential fatty acids are necessary for growth and for the overall health of the blood vessels and nerves. Based on our experience with our patients, we believe that African Americans need more essential fatty acids than people of other races.

Consider the Evidence

- *HEART DISEASE.* Omega-3 fatty acids help to thin the blood and prevent the formation of blood clots that can cause heart attack. Studies have shown that omega-3 fatty acids can lower total cholesterol and triglyceride levels in people who also cut back on saturated fat. Other studies by the National Heart and Lung Institute have shown that eating as little as 1 gram of omega-3 fatty acids daily may reduce the risk of cardiovascular disease by as much as 40 percent.

- *STROKE.* Eating fish can lower your risk of stroke. A long-term Dutch study found that men who ate more than 20 grams (about 0.67 ounce) of fish per day had a lower risk of stroke than those who ate less fish.

- *CANCER.* A number of animal studies have shown that omega-3 fatty acids can delay the onset of tumors and decrease the rate of growth, size, and number of tumors that develop in research animals. It is worth noting that other studies have found that other types of fat (especially saturated fats) can increase tumor growth.

- *ARTHRITIS.* Omega-3 fatty acids can help to reduce the pain and inflammation associated with some types of arthritis. Several studies found that people with rheumatoid arthritis found relief when they took omega-3 fatty acid supplements in addition to their nonsteroid anti-inflammatory drugs.

- *DIABETES.* A Dutch study found that older people (those sixty-four to eighty-seven) who ate fish regularly for three years were less likely to develop glucose intolerance and diabetes than those who consumed less fish.

Omega-3 fatty acid (or linolenic acid) is found in flaxseed, soybean, canola, pumpkin, and walnut oils. Omega-6 fatty acid (linoleic acid) is found in soybean, safflower, sunflower, corn, wheat germ, and sesame oils.

Salmon, mackerel, herring, and sardines are good sources of fish oil because they have the highest fat content and provide more omega-3 factors than other fish. For example, salmon contains about ten times more omega-3 fatty acids than cod, a low-fat fish.

R~x~ for Health

- Take 1 gram of omega-3 fish oil three times a day and 500 milligrams of omega-6 three times a day at the same time.

  NOTE: *Do not take omega-3 supplements if you take a blood-thinning drug or use aspirin daily without first consulting your physician. High amounts of omega-3 fatty acids may cause bleeding or hemorrhagic stroke.*

L-Glutamine

The amino acid L-glutamine is found in animal and vegetable proteins; it is also found in high concentrations in the human brain, where it is essential for cerebral function. It allows the body to increase its levels of growth hormone, in addition to speeding the body's repair of the digestive tract. L-glutamine has been used in the treatment of fatigue, peptic ulcers, impotence, parkinsonism, muscular dystrophy, mental retardation, obesity, and alcoholism.

Consider the Evidence

- *ALCOHOLISM.* Studies have found that L-glutamine decreases the craving for alcohol. (Glutamic acid should not be substituted for L-glutamine in the treatment of alcoholism; it does not work as well.)

- *OBESITY.* L-glutamine reduces the craving for sugar and carbohydrates, making it useful in the treatment of obesity.

L-glutamine, like other amino acids, is available in multivitamin formulas, food supplements, protein mixtures, or amino acid formulas. It can be purchased in capsule, tablet, or powder form.

R$_x$ for Health
- Take 1 gram three times a day.

L-Cysteine

This sulfur-containing amino acid is used by the liver and the immune system to detoxify chemicals; it is also used in a number of metabolic processes.

Consider the Evidence

- *ANTIOXIDANT PROTECTOR.* L-cysteine stabilizes the cell membrane, reducing the hazards of smoking cigarettes and drinking alcohol. It does this by helping to neutralize the aldehydes produced as a by-product of the metabolism of alcohol, fats, and air pollution.

- *HEAVY METALS.* L-cysteine tends to bind with heavy metals (such as lead, mercury, and cadmium), helping the body eliminate these toxins before they cause damage.

L-cysteine, like other amino acids, is available in multivitamin formulas, food supplements, protein mixtures, or amino acid formulas. It can be purchased in capsule, tablet, or powder form.

R$_x$ for Health

- Take 500 milligrams daily in divided doses.
  NOTE: Take amino acids on an empty stomach for best absorption.

HOW MUCH IS ENOUGH?

And how much is too much? To help answer these questions, more than forty years ago the U.S. Food and Nutrition Board set out to determine daily amounts of vitamins necessary to prevent disease. The federal government has established recommended dietary allowances (RDAs) for essential nutrients, using information provided by the Food and Nutrition Board of the National Academy of Sciences National Research Council. The RDAs vary with age and sex, though in an attempt to simplify matters, a single RDA is used on food labels.

RDAs are based on whether a nutrient is essential for the body's health, and on the amount required to prevent deficiency and disease. RDAs are designed to prevent nutritional disease, not to achieve optimal health. That's why many experts recommend that people take vitamins and minerals at higher, therapeutic levels to prevent or manage various ailments or diseases. Instead of thinking of minimum amounts necessary to prevent disease, we should think of Optimum Daily Allowance to promote and enhance health.

Taking vitamins and nutritional supplements to meet the RDAs is not harmful, but self-diagnosing and taking megadoses of specific vitamins can be. When the body encounters large doses of water-soluble vitamins, the excess that the body can't use is simply excreted in the urine. However, fat-soluble vitamins can accumulate in the body and cause potential health problems. There is an appropriate range of vitamin intake, and consuming too little or too much of some nutrients can be dangerous.

In 1994, the FDA revised its nutrition labeling program and

replaced the RDAs with Daily Values (DVs) for vitamins, minerals, and other nutrients. Food labels now state the percentage of the DV for selected vitamins and minerals.

FINDING A QUALIFIED NUTRITIONIST

If you have special nutritional needs, or want help to design a regimen of nutritional supplements to help manage your specific health needs, you may want to consult a nutrition counselor. For information on finding a qualified nutritionist and publications on nutrition, see page 318.

10
▼

Líving Clean

Minimizing Your Environmental Risks

We live in a toxic world. The environment around us contains both visible and invisible hazards that can take their toll on our health. A glass of water may appear clear and mountain-spring pure, but it may actually contain dangerous levels of pesticides or heavy metals. The food we eat may taste fresh and free of off-flavors or chemical residue, while it may in fact contain potentially cancer-causing additives. It can be difficult to strike an appropriate balance when talking about environmental risks: Some people disregard risks they cannot see and others become paranoid and excessively fearful of them. Neither ignorance nor fear is in our best interest. We need to understand the risks we face in our daily lives and take steps to minimize our exposures to those toxins we can avoid.

While environmental health risks affect all of us, they tend to affect African Americans more than many other groups. According to the U.S. Environmental Protection Agency, African Americans and other people of color suffer disproportionately from exposure to dust, soot, carbon monoxide, ozone, sulfur, sulfur dioxide, lead, and other environmental hazards, both at home and in the workplace. This means that we must put forth special effort to detect and minimize our exposure to these risks.

In order to do this, we must resist the temptation to accept the Western magic-bullet mentality. We cannot assume that if one chemical causes a problem with the environment, we will be able to come up with another that can reverse the damage and make things right.

Instead of looking for a chemical quick fix, we need to view the environment holistically, just as we view our bodies holistically.

As individuals, we can take steps to protect the environment, but we must also take steps to protect the internal environment in our bodies. Chronic exposure to environmental toxins will take its toll on our health; some ill effects may be felt in the short term, while others may take twenty or thirty years to show up. These repeated chemical insults may manifest themselves as mild symptoms or as severe—or even fatal—health problems.

▼▼▼▼▼▼▼▼▼▼▼▼▼▼▼▼▼▼▼▼▼▼▼▼▼

ARE YOU BEING POISONED?

There can be many symptoms of chemical toxicity, but some of the most common ones include:

- Headache

- Memory loss

- Problems with concentration

- Confusion

- Fatigue

- Mood swings

- Nervousness

- Loss of sex drive

- Skin rashes

- Nausea

- Coughing and wheezing

- Anorexia

- Edema

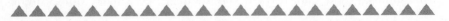

We encourage all of our patients to take an environmental inventory of their toxic exposures. When we assess the health of our patients, we look for what we refer to as "the unhealthy trinity"—toxic food, toxic water, and toxic energy. No one can avoid exposure to all industrial chemicals and toxins, but there are steps we can take to reduce our risks.

TOXIC FOOD

As a general rule, the more processed the food, the more toxic the food. Food manufacturers use more than three thousand different food additives in processed and packaged foods. In addition to heaping helpings of salt and sugar, manufacturers add emulsifiers and buffers, artificial flavors and colors, and literally hundreds of chemicals designed to preserve, enhance, or otherwise alter the food from the way Mother Nature made it. Some coffee creamers, candies, and other foods are actually made entirely of man-made chemicals.

If you are like the average American, you consume nearly 150 pounds of these food additives each year. As an African American, you may consume even more, since we tend to eat more processed foods than people of other races. These additives can cause health problems, especially among chemically sensitive individuals. In addition, they may contribute to the high rate of cancer in the United States. Consider that the nitrites and nitrates added to foods can form carcinogenic nitrosamines in our bodies, and sulfites, which are commonly used in food to prevent spoilage and discoloration, can cause allergic reactions in some people. We have had a number of patients whose vague neurological symptoms were traced back to sensitivity to aspartame, or Nutrasweet. (Aspartame breaks down into formaldehyde in the body.) In addition, some food additives—such as Red Dye #2, cyclamates, and cobalt sulfate—were once considered safe but later withdrawn from the market.

Intentional food additives must be listed as ingredients on product labels, but as many as twelve thousand additional chemicals contaminate our foods at various stages of growing, harvesting, and packaging. The pesticides sprayed on foods, the antibiotics and hormones fed to the animals that produce the food, and the chemicals in the water used to process the food can all contribute to the toxicity of food.

Another problem is that chemicals that may not pose a threat individually may combine with others and form new, more dangerous chemicals. The best way to avoid toxins in food is to eat those foods our ancestors ate—wholesome, natural foods free of pesticides, hormones, and antibiotics. Give preference to those grown locally, since they are less likely to require the use of preservatives.

Whenever possible look for range-fed animals. Not only do range-fed animals have fewer chemical contaminants, but they also have more health-enhancing fatty acids. For example, range-fed chickens have more omega-3 fatty acids than those grown in a crowded chicken coop.

You can minimize your exposure to chemicals by buying whole foods that have been grown organically. These foods are not necessarily free of all chemical residues—no farmer can make that promise—but it does mean that farmers have avoided the use of chemicals during growing. Of course, pesticides that had been applied to previous crops may remain in the soil, and some plants absorb chemicals from contaminated water. Even organic foods can contain dangerous chemicals, though certainly in much smaller quantities than conventionally grown produce.

In addition, sometimes produce is mislabeled (either intentionally or accidentally). We have known people who loved mangoes and shopped at a particular market because they were labeled "organically grown." A friend from the Food Inspection Service at the U.S. Department of Agriculture told us that the mangoes have been dipped in insecticide. She said, "No matter what the sticker says, we dip those things when they come into the country. We don't want to let any insects in here." Even if produce is organically grown overseas, it may be chemically treated before it is imported and sold. That's another good reason to wash all produce thoroughly—including organic produce—before eating it or serving it to your family. It's also a good reason to choose domestically grown produce if it is available.

Since the foods we eat can either nourish or poison our bodies, we have detailed discussions with our patients about the foods they eat. Unfortunately, many of our patients report that they enjoy (too often) the high-fat, high-sodium, high-sugar foods from fast-food places.

These foods may be fast and relatively cheap, but they are poison to the body. Why? Fast-food places offer a diet of white bread (minimal nutritional value); burgers, fries, and chicken cooked in superheated oils (which become carcinogenic and depleted of vitamin E due to the high temperatures); and fatty sauces. One of the best things you can do for yourself is to stop eating at fast-food restaurants.

℞ FOR HEALTH

- Buy organic foods when possible.

- Buy range-fed animals when possible.

- Minimize your use of processed foods.

- Avoid the food additives listed below.

▼▼▼▼▼▼▼▼▼▼▼▼▼▼▼▼▼▼▼▼▼▼▼▼▼▼

THE FOOD ADDITIVE MOST WANTED (AND LEAST WANTED) LIST

Additives to Avoid
Artificial colors
Sodium nitrite and nitrate
Butylate hydroxytoluene (BHT)
Saccharin
Sulfites (especially sodium bisulfite)
Sulfur dioxide
Monosodium glutamate (MSG)
Brominated vegetable oil (BVO)
Hydrogenated vegetable oils
Natural flavorings
Additives to Limit
Butylate hydroxyanisole (BHA)
Sugars (sucrose, dextrose, corn syrup)
Artificial flavorings
Prophy gallate
Salt

Aspartame
Caffeine
Propylene glycol
Gums
Xylitol
Aluminum salts

Probably Safe

Vitamins A, C, and E
Beta-carotene or carotene
Carrageenan
Annatto
Citric acid, sorbic acid, lactic acid
Alginates
Iron, zinc, and other minerals
Glycerin (mono- and diglycerides)
Gelatin
Pectin
Calcium propionate
Polysorbate 60, 65, 80
Sorbitol
Sodium benzoate
Lecithin
Lactose
Vanillin
Potassium sorbate

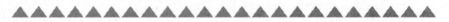

TOXIC WATER

Water is essential for life and health; it literally washes toxins out of our bodies. Unfortunately, we have found that African Americans rarely drink enough water. Some of our patients tell us that they avoid water (and drink sugared sodas or sodas laced with artificial sweeteners instead) because they fear their water is polluted. In most cases, we would rather see people drink eight glasses of tap water than two glasses of soda or cola. Once people have committed to drinking enough water, then we can discuss water quality.

As we mentioned before, we recommend that you take your weight in pounds and divide that number in half to determine the ideal number of ounces of water you should drink a day. For example, if you weigh 150 pounds, you should drink 75 ounces of water. For most people the ideal is between 60 and 90 ounces. (For more information on drinking water, see page 100.)

You may lose your thirst when you think of all the substances that can contaminate water—microorganisms (such as bacteria and viruses), dissolved solids (such as nitrates, fluoride, and mineral salts), particulate matter (such as dirt, rust, and heavy metals), and volatile chemicals (such as pesticides). Many municipalities add chlorine to the water supply to wipe out the microorganisms and filter the water to catch the rest. (We appreciate concern about the carcinogenic properties of chlorine, which is why we recommend filtered water.)

This bleach-and-filter approach works reasonably well in most areas, but you can minimize your exposure to some toxins by filtering or purifying water. Reverse osmosis filter systems do an excellent job, but they can be expensive and require good water pressure. (They also take up a lot of room under the sink.) Carbon block filters can do a good job as well, and they are usually cheaper and smaller. If you don't feel comfortable drinking from your public water system—even with a filter—then buy bottled water by the gallon from the health food store or supermarket.

If you live in an area supplied by a well rather than a municipal water system, have your water tested—and then retested every three to five years. Agricultural runoff can pollute the subterranean water source, making well water just as toxic as—or more toxic than—public water.

During a period of detoxification, some people prefer to drink distilled water (water with all minerals removed), but distilled water should be used as drinking water for only a week or two at a time. Some doctors and nutritionists believe that distilled water can contribute to a deficiency of calcium and magnesium by drawing these minerals out of the body. To our knowledge, this theory has never been proven, but we still discourage the long-term use of distilled water unless you are taking mineral supplements or have been directed to do so by your health care practitioner.

R_X for Health

- Drink plenty of water. (Take your weight in pounds and divide by two; that is the ideal number of ounces.)

- Use a reverse osmosis filter for your tap water.

- Test your water quality if your water comes from a well or if your municipal water has a strange taste, smell, or appearance. Retest every three to five years as needed.

▼▼▼▼▼▼▼▼▼▼▼▼▼▼▼▼▼▼▼▼▼▼▼▼▼▼

THE AIR YOU BREATHE MAY BE HAZARDOUS TO YOUR HEALTH

You don't have much choice: You have to breathe. But in certain conditions, a big breath of air can result in a big dose of pollutants. Often the air inside your home or workplace may be more toxic than the outside air. Why? Outside the pollution has a chance to dissipate into the air; inside the new, airtight buildings where we live and work, we trap the toxic gases in the interior environment.

We have found that a disproportionate number of African Americans experience "sick building syndrome" and other health problems associated with toxic indoor air. Though it is an unproven hypothesis, we suspect that underlying nutritional problems make blacks more susceptible to illness of all kinds, including air-related illness.

Common indoor pollutants to watch out for include hydrocarbon fuel (burning coal, natural gas, or gasoline), pesticides and insecticides, cleaning fluids, paints, adhesives, glues, solvents, plastics, secondary smoke, fireplace smoke, aerosol sprays, and even dust, which can carry mites, molds, bacteria, and pollens.

Another risk is radon gas, an odorless, invisible, radioactive gas that can seep into your home through the foundation, basement, and water supply. Radon can damage the lungs; it is considered the second leading cause of lung cancer after smoking. For more information on indoor air quality, contact the U.S. Environmental Protection Agency at (202) 233-9340.

▲▲▲▲▲▲▲▲▲▲▲▲▲▲▲▲▲▲▲▲▲▲▲▲▲▲▲▲

TOXIC ENERGY

When patients complain of headaches, fatigue, memory loss, and other vague symptoms, one of the things we ask them about is their exposure to electric appliances—electric blankets, hair dryers, computers, and so forth. We believe that the electromagnetic fields caused by these appliances can have a subtle but meaningful impact on health.

When assessing the health impact of exposure to electromagnetic fields, you must realize that there are two main types of electromagnetic radiation:

- **Ionizing Radiation** (including X rays, gamma rays, and nuclear radiation). This type of radiation is powerful enough to change the structure of atoms and molecules; it can directly affect cell division.

- **Nonionizing Radiation** (electromagnetic radiation below 300 hertz or cycles per second, including the 60-hertz currents used by residential and office appliances). This type of radiation can't directly alter cell structure, but it can generate heat and vibration.

While virtually everyone agrees that ionizing radiation causes serious health problems, there is more controversy surrounding the detrimental effects of nonionizing radiation. However, a growing body of evidence suggests that ongoing exposure to electro-pollution in the form of nonionizing radiation can cause a number of health problems.

Electromagnetic fields are measured in a unit known as a gauss. The intensity of the electromagnetic field near humming high-voltage power lines and near high-current appliances often equals 1 gauss. Researchers have found that people exposed to a 1-gauss field have compromised short-term memory that those not exposed to the radiation don't exhibit. People living near high-voltage power lines have complained about headaches, memory loss, fatigue, and weakness. Cattle grazing near high-voltage lines produced less milk and gave birth to calves with an increased number of birth defects. Similarly, pregnant women who sleep under electric blankets have been found to have a higher rate of miscarriages than other women. Other studies have suggested that electricians, electronic technicians, and utility linemen experience a greater risk of brain tumors than people who aren't exposed to electromagnetic fields for prolonged periods of time.

When assessing the risk of nonionizing radiation, remember that our bodies rely on electrical pulses to power reactions in our muscles, nerves, and cells. (Just think of the surge of electricity from the paddles used to resuscitate heart attack patients.) Many of the functions performed by our bodies depend on the electrical currents constantly moving through and across the cell membranes. In fact, our bodies are surrounded by a measurable electromagnetic field and alive with an unmeasurable but no less real energy or life force.

In fact, the Earth itself vibrates with an electromagnetic pulse equal to about 10 hertz (which, coincidentally, is equal to the level of electromagnetic activity in the human brain during rest). Many appliances and power lines operate in the range of 45 to 70 hertz, close enough to the Earth's vibration and the vibration of the human body that it may agitate or stimulate our biocycles, causing stress, fatigue, and a reduced resistance to disease. There is much we don't know, but researchers have shown that magnetic fields affect the pineal gland, which pumps out serotonin and melatonin and plays a critical role in the endocrine system.

Other animals rely on electromagnetic fields to understand their environment. Many birds, insects, reptiles, and sea creatures use the Earth's electromagnetic fields to establish their sense of direction. Consider the behavior changes in animals when they "sense" an oncoming earthquake or severe changes in weather by noting changes in the electromagnetic fields. Keeping this in mind, it does not seem far-fetched to believe that environmental electromagnetic fields can and do affect our health.

℞ FOR HEALTH

- Ground yourself for a few minutes every day. The Earth itself can be very useful in balancing electromagnetism. Step outside barefoot and sink your toes in the soil. Feel the Earth; relax. This will help clear your body of unneeded electricity.

- Minimize your use of electric appliances. If you can allow your hair to air dry instead of standing under a hair dryer, do it. If you can shave with a blade razor instead of an electric razor, do it. You get the idea.

- Keep your appliances at arm's length. You can reduce your exposure to magnetic fields by positioning yourself a few feet away from them when they are in use. (Putting the alarm clock more than an arm's length away will not only reduce your exposure to electromagnetic fields, but it will help you wake up by forcing you to drag yourself out of bed to turn off the alarm.) If you work with a computer or other electric office equipment for hours at home or in the office, make it a point to keep the machines at arm's length and to avoid exposure to the back of the machines (most of the radiation escapes from the back).

▼▼▼▼▼▼▼▼▼▼▼▼▼▼▼▼▼▼▼▼▼▼▼

DR. SINGLETON'S ELECTRIC BLANKET

I used to sleep with an old and inefficient electric blanket. Then I developed a number of chronic problems, including severe fatigue, headaches, a skin rash, ridges in my fingernails, and gastrointestinal symptoms. I thought about the advice I would give my own patients and decided to learn more about electromagnetic fields.

I did a lot of reading and found out that electromagnetic fields can inhibit melatonin release, which can interfere with sleep and cause fatigue. It's no wonder that I felt warm but not well rested. I bought a meter to measure the electromagnetic fields in my home; the field around the blanket was in excess of one gauss. I threw away the electric blanket, convinced I suffered from electromagnetic radiation toxicity. My symptoms cleared up within three months. Now if I feel cold at night, I warm up the old-fashioned way: I reach for another blanket.

▲▲▲▲▲▲▲▲▲▲▲▲▲▲▲▲▲▲▲▲▲▲▲▲

GET THE LEAD OUT

Lead poisoning poses a special risk to African American children, who are exposed to lead much more often than white children. This toxic metal—which can contaminate paint, water, oil, and air—is the leading cause of environmental poisoning to children.

Lead can accumulate in the body, damaging the nervous system, kidneys, and blood. It can cause behavioral and developmental problems, as well as lower IQ. In extreme cases, lead poisoning can cause death.

The problem is most severe in children under age six (who are more likely to eat paint chips or put their hands in their mouths). This generation of our children faces a lesser risk than previous generations due to restrictions on the use of lead in paint and gasoline. Still, lead can pose a serious risk, especially if you live in the inner city or in a house built before 1978. Most dishes and glassware made in the United States are free of lead, but ceramics made abroad have been known to contain high levels of lead.

We recommend that you have your children tested for lead at nine to twelve months of age and again at twenty-four months. If you live in an older home or a high-risk area, ask about a lead retest during your child's annual checkup. Be sure your child's diet includes plenty of iron, calcium, and protein, since deficiencies in these nutrients can increase a child's absorption of lead. For more information about lead, contact the National Lead Information Center hotline at (800) LEAD-FYI or the Centers for Disease Control at (404) 488-7330.

PART 3

Healing Ourselves

11

Overcoming Our Addictions

Giving Up Alcohol, Drugs, and Tobacco

Addictions—whether to alcohol, drugs, or nicotine—involve more than a physical dependence on a chemical high. While we do not deny the biochemistry of addiction and we acknowledge that some people respond well to antidepressants and other drugs to realign the body's chemistry, we believe that the addict's spiritual or psychological cravings are even more important than the physical ones.

At their core, addictive behaviors involve an attempt to relieve pain without experiencing real healing. In almost every case we have seen—and we have seen thousands of addicts during our careers—the addicted person perceives himself as being hurt, violated, or abused in some way, whether physical, emotional, sexual, or racial. The person holds on to the pain and develops a resentment about the experience; in many cases, the pain is then used as an excuse for abusing alcohol, drugs, or nicotine.

When a person hangs on to the pain and uses it to justify a self-centered, self-absorbed, self-destructive approach to life, we say they suffer from a "victim mentality." In such cases, the addicts feel entitled to do what they want because they have been victimized. Victim mentality is the basis of almost every hard-core addiction we have seen.

An example of someone who overcame his addiction when he gave up his victim mentality was a twenty-year-old homeless man who was addicted to cocaine. He had lived a hard life; in fact, he had been victimized by people who should have loved him. His reaction to his situation was self-pity, bitterness, and resentment. We recommended that he seek help from Narcotics Anonymous because the program gently but systematically confronts the person with their victim mentality. This man hung in throughout the process and found fellowship and support from the group. He was able to overcome his addiction because he was able to overcome his victim mentality.

Healing involves taking responsibility for our actions. While we're not responsible for the things that have happened to us, we are responsible for our responses to those experiences. If we are holding on to resentment, we can let go of it; we must stop using the past to justify the present. Something may have happened to you twenty-five years ago that wounded you deeply, but if you still feel victimized by that experience a quarter century later and use it as an excuse for an addiction, you have become a victim of your own flawed thinking. To heal, you must forgive your victimizers and let go of bitterness; you must move forward instead of feeling emotionally trapped in the episode that caused your pain.

To heal the pain, you do not necessarily need to go back and relive it. What you need to do is confront the maladaptive way you have chosen to react to your pain. You can heal yourself and overcome your addiction without fully understanding the pain. Some psychoanalysts may tell you that you need to go back and rediscover the pain to heal yourself, but we believe the most important issue is to start moving forward.

To overcome an addiction, the patient must realize that they have a choice and they have the power to choose health. The natural remedies and methods of healing we will describe in the rest of this chapter can help the addicted person deal with the physical changes associated with giving up an addiction. However, these techniques will be successful only if the person has reached the point of truth and made a conscious decision that the time has come to be healed. In some cases, the task may be easier with help from a medical professional; we encourage you to work with a physician or practitioner with experience in addiction treatment if you think such a person will help you overcome your addiction.

▼▼▼▼▼▼▼▼▼▼▼▼▼▼▼▼▼▼▼▼▼▼

DR. SINGLETON ON THE POOLSIDE PARABLE

It can be very difficult to get a "victim" to surrender his or her status as victim. After all, victims get a lot of attention (they need to be taken care of) and they don't have to take full responsibility for their actions (they have an excuse for all their shortcomings). As long as an addict is entrenched in this type of thinking, there is little we can do to break the addiction because the addict does not understand that he has the power to help himself.

In those patients who recognize that they have some control over the choices they make in their lives, I have had a lot of success building a discussion around a passage in the Bible, John 5:1-14. Though most of our African American patients have a Christian background, we don't use the reading as a Christian text, but rather as a text that contains certain illustrations that may prove useful.

I start by simply reading the story of the healing at the pool:

Some time later, Jesus went up to Jerusalem for a feast of the Jews. Now there is in Jerusalem near the Sheep Gate a pool, which in Aramaic is called Bethesda and which is surrounded by five covered colonnades. Here a great number of disabled people used to lie—the blind, the lame, the paralyzed. One who was there had been an invalid for thirty-eight years. When Jesus saw him lying there and learned that he had been in this condition for a long time, he asked him, "Do you want to get well?"

"Sir," the invalid replied, "I have no one to help me into the pool when the water is stirred. While I am trying to get in, someone else goes down ahead of me."

Then Jesus said to him, "Get up! Pick up your mat and walk." At once the man was cured; he picked up his mat and walked. . . . Later, Jesus found him at the temple and said to him, "See, you are well again. Stop sinning or something worse may happen to you."

JOHN 5:1-14 (NEW INTERNATIONAL VERSION)

After the reading, we discuss the meaning of the story, and several things become clear: In order to become well, we must stop making excuses and choose to be healed; we must stop making excuses and waiting for someone to help us into the water and walk for ourselves.

While this parable doesn't work for every patient, it's amazing how often it helps people work through their narcisism and self-pity to the point that they can experience the insight that they have been making excuses and justifying their behavior inappropriately.

▲▲▲▲▲▲▲▲▲▲▲▲▲▲▲▲▲▲▲▲▲▲▲▲▲▲

SETTING YOURSELF FREE

To successfully overcome our addictions, we must detoxify our bodies and change our abusive habits. This process is more complex than it may sound, since we live in an addictive culture and we use any number of substances (both legal and illegal) to alter our mood. Rather than trying to understand our feelings and their causes, we use stimulants or sedatives to change the feelings that make us uncomfortable. We need to view our emotions holistically; we need to explore the depths of our feelings rather than simply medicating the symptoms of emotional stress.

Before launching into a program of alcohol, drug, or nicotine detoxification, we recommend that you make a plan. You may want to ask for help from a doctor, therapist, or close friend who will be able to provide support during the difficult process of withdrawal. With any kind of addictive problem, there are several phases you must pass through:

- **Admit your addiction.** Before you can fight an addiction you must admit you are an addict. Only after you acknowledge the addiction can you commit to changing your behavior. Unfortunately, it often takes a serious illness or crisis to bring an addict to this point of transformation, but there is little that one person can do to make another want to be healthy.

- **Detoxify your body.** This initial period of withdrawal can last for several days or weeks. During this period, your body is learning how to function without the drug, and the body is releasing the stored chemicals that build up during the period of abuse.

- **Repattern your behavior.** You need to learn how to live without the substance you crave. It takes willpower—a lot of willpower—to make a commitment to overcome an addiction. At this point, it is essential to develop new behavior patterns and to avoid situations that can tempt you to succumb to your self-destructive old patterns.

- **Nourish your body.** During the period of detoxification and recovery, you need to nourish your body by eating wholesome foods and taking appropriate nutritional supplements. Drink a lot of water to help flush toxins from the body. Eat high-fiber foods to draw toxins out of the colon. Many people find fasting helpful during detoxification; for more information, see Chapter 6 on page 103.

▼▼▼▼▼▼▼▼▼▼▼▼▼▼▼▼▼▼▼▼▼▼▼▼▼▼▼

DR. WALKER AND THE SPIRITUAL ASPECT OF ADDICTION

Addiction is part of the human condition. Every culture that has been studied, with the exception of several Eskimo tribes, has included people who suffer from addiction. For many of these people, I suspect that the addiction is an attempt to bypass the issues of this world in an attempt to become closer to God. Of course, this approach doesn't work and the addict becomes lost in an illusion. It seems that God has arranged things so that we come to know Him through our actions and deeds and through being responsible for our own self-management. Only by being responsible for our individual lives will we build what is required to recognize the God that is within us and within the universe. Sobriety starts with speaking your truth to yourself, to those you trust, and to God. By discovering your truth, you can know yourself and your God.

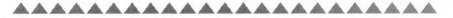

Alcohol Addiction

One hundred years ago, African Americans had the lowest death rate due to alcoholism of any racial or ethnic group in the country. In fact, alcoholism among African Americans was so unusual that some people considered us immune from its scourge. As we now know all too well, this is not the case.

African Americans suffer disproportionately from alcoholism and its complications. African Americans tend to start drinking at an earlier age compared to people of other races. Liver disease and its complications are the ninth leading cause of death in the United States, and the death rate for blacks is almost twice that of whites. Each year, some forty thousand people die due to cirrhosis of the liver, a disease caused by alcohol abuse.

If you consume enough alcohol, it will damage your body—period. Drinking 80 grams of alcohol—the amount found in a six-pack of beer, five 6-ounce glasses of wine, or five martinis—is enough to damage the liver and pancreas if you drink on a daily basis. The liver is affected because it is the only organ that metabolizes alcohol. (Fully 95 percent of alcohol is metabolized by the liver; the remaining 5 percent is excreted through sweat, urine, and breathing.) In the body, alcohol is converted into fat rather than glucose or glycogen for energy. This fat irritates the liver, resulting in cirrhosis, a process of swelling, scarring, and shriveling as the disease progresses. In the treatment of alcoholism, many doctors refer to the law of sevens: Drinking 80 grams of alcohol or more a day will cause cirrhosis of the liver in seven years, acute pancreatitis in seven more years, and death within seven years after that. Of course, some people may suffer harmful effects at lower amounts, but this is a general rule of thumb.

Alcohol is a toxin and when ingested it systematically destroys the body. Consider the evidence:

- Alcohol inhibits the liver's production of digestive enzymes and interferes with the body's ability to absorb vitamins A, D, E, and K, as well as the B vitamins.

- Alcohol irritates the lining of the gastrointestinal tract, including the esophagus, stomach, and upper small intestine. It increases the production of hydrochloric acid in the stomach, causing stomach inflammation and abdominal pain.

- Alcohol kills brain cells. Alcohol crosses the blood-brain barrier and damages the brain tissues, sometimes resulting in brain damage and psychological or behavior problems.

- Alcohol can cause painful nerve inflammation or a condition known as polyneuritis. (This is especially common when there is a deficiency in B vitamins.)

- Alcohol contributes to diabetes and hypoglycemia because chronic use can weaken glucose tolerance. Alcohol is a simple sugar.

Some recent studies have shown that there can be cardiovascular benefits associated with *moderate* alcohol consumption, but an alcoholic by definition cannot drink moderately. Alcoholism may be triggered by a genetic predisposition, a metabolic problem, an allergy, or some other factor. Whatever the cause, the first step toward recovery is to admit the problem and seek help.

We have found very few people can quit drinking without assistance. It is often difficult to separate the psychological and spiritual issues from the physical dependency on alcohol. The challenge is to reclaim your will, and we often need the support of others in order to do this. In addition, you will need to consult a medical professional if you think you will need tranquilizers or other prescription drugs to make it through the period of detoxification. Hospitalization may be necessary for acute alcohol withdrawal. (When looking for a doctor with experience and expertise in alcoholism, consider those with certification from the American Society of Addiction Medicine, 4601 N. Park Ave., Suite 101, Chevy Chase, MD 20815, (301) 656-3920.)

The experience of detoxification varies, depending on how much and how long you have been drinking. Most people feel tense and irritable, often with a headache, for the first few days of withdrawal. More advanced alcoholics may experience seizures and neurological symptoms, which should be cared for by a professional.

During detoxification, avoid exposing yourself to alcohol; don't spend time with drinking buddies or attend parties where alcohol will be served. During the times you used to drink or feel tempted to drink, exercise or go for a walk. If you feel you might indulge, call a friend and ask for help; don't go it alone.

For the first few days of detoxification, dramatically increase your protein consumption by eating more fish, chicken, salmon, turkey, and plant proteins. In addition, consume an alkaline liquid diet—water, diluted fruit and vegetable juices, broths, and herbal teas; teas made with the herbs chamomile, peppermint, skullcap, and valerian can be quite soothing. Avoid sugars, refined foods, and dairy products. Drink at least 64 ounces of water a day; drinking water throughout the day can help flush toxins from the body, speeding the period of detoxification. (Eat lots of small meals; this is preferable to fewer large meals.)

To replace the nutrients lost during the days you used alcohol, we recommend you take a good multiple vitamin/mineral supplement. In addition, we tell our patients to take extra zinc (50 milligrams), calcium (5000 milligrams), magnesium (1000 milligrams), and thiamine (25 milligrams). (Alcoholics tend to develop a thiamine deficiency—also known as beriberi—because alcohol blocks thiamine absorption in the intestine.) To help maintain a steady blood sugar level, which can help minimize cravings for alcohol, we recommend an additional chromium (200 micrograms daily) for the first three months of sobriety.

R_x for Health

- Seek help from Alcoholics Anonymous (AA), Rational Recovery (RR), Secular Organizations for Sobriety (SOS), or another support network. In addition to the issues of physical dependence, there are underlying issues that caused the alcoholic to begin drinking, and these issues need to be explored.

- To help reduce the cravings for alcohol, take 250 to 500 milligrams of L-glutamine twice a day, and 25 milligrams of vitamin B_6 three or four times a day. Take these supplements for four to six weeks, then reduce the dosage by half and take them for two more weeks. If cravings persist, use supplements as needed and consult a medical professional.

- Contact an acupuncturist with expertise in managing addictions. Acupuncture can be quite effective in reducing cravings.

▼▼▼▼▼▼▼▼▼▼▼▼▼▼▼▼▼▼▼▼▼▼▼

Is AA for You?

Only you can decide whether you want to give AA a try. Here are some questions to answer honestly. If you answer Yes to four or more questions, you may be a problem drinker. Remember, there is no disgrace in facing up to the fact that you have a problem.

1. Have you ever decided to stop drinking for a week or so but lasted only for a couple of days?

2. Do you wish people would mind their own business about your drinking—stop telling you what to do?

3. Have you ever switched from one kind of drink to another in the hope that this would keep you from getting drunk?

4. Have you had to have an eye-opener upon awakening during the past year?

5. Do you envy people who can drink without getting into trouble?

6. Have you had problems connected with drinking during the past year?

7. Has your drinking caused trouble at home?

8. Do you ever try to get "extra" drinks at a party because you do not get enough?

9. Do you tell yourself you can stop drinking any time you want to even though you keep getting drunk when you don't mean to?

10. Have you missed days of work or school because of drinking?

11. Do you have "blackouts"?

12. Have you ever felt that your life would be better if you did not drink?

Reprinted with the permission of Alcoholics Anonymous World Services, Inc.

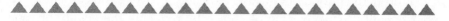

Drug Addiction

Drug abuse has ravaged our communities and destroyed many African American lives. To the individual hooked on a drug—whether an illegal drug, a prescription medication, or an over-the-counter drug—the addiction can undermine personal relationships, cause financial ruin, and even result in death.

If you use drugs recreationally, you need to examine your behavior. You may not be addicted, but you should assess the reasons you feel compelled to experiment with drugs in the first place. A support group or individual counseling can prove helpful in figuring out the motives and emotions behind your actions.

Recreational drug users—those who use drugs no more than once or twice a month and who often go three months without using drugs—and recovering addicts often respond well to good nutritional support. Hard-core drug addictions usually must be handled on an inpatient basis, followed up with a regimen of natural treatments.

If you use drugs with any regularity, you may need to consult with a doctor before stopping "cold turkey." Abruptly discontinuing the use of sedatives, stimulants, or narcotics can result in potentially dangerous side effects. (Sedative withdrawal can cause seizures, stimulant withdrawal can cause depression, and narcotic withdrawal can cause sweating, abdominal pain, insomnia, and diarrhea, among other symptoms.) In some cases, a physician may prescribe tranquilizers or other medications for a short period of time to help with the withdrawal period.

Detoxification is a crucial step in freeing yourself from an addiction. Herbs can be quite helpful in removing drug-related toxins from the body, especially during the first four to six weeks of sobriety. Many manufacturers of herbal treatments offer commercial detoxification formulas; Twin Labs offers an excellent formula that can be helpful in minimizing cravings and cleanse the body at an accelerated rate. In your health food store, look for commercially prepared products containing red clover and goldenseal; both herbs are helpful in liver detoxification. Chlorophyll, either taken as a liquid or in tablet form, can help to rejuvenate and purify the body. Follow package directions for dosage information.

During the period of detoxification and recovery, you can minimize your cravings for your drug of choice by reducing the acidity of your diet and increasing the alkalinity. Avoid acid-forming dairy products, refined flours, and sugar, and replace them with alkaline-promoting fruits and vegetables. The cravings should pass within several months, but this more healthful diet should be continued for life!

R̪ for Health

- Seek help from Narcotics Anonymous or another support network. In addition to the issues of physical dependence, there are underlying issues that caused the addict to use drugs, and these issues need to be explored.

- Use commercially prepared herbal products containing red clover and goldenseal, which help with detoxification. Follow package directions. These herbal treatments can be used for four to six weeks.

- Contact an acupuncturist with expertise in managing addictions.

- For the first four to six weeks of sobriety, supplement your diet with additional vitamins and minerals. In addition to taking a good multiple vitamin/mineral supplement, we recommend the following:

Vitamin C (2 grams)
Vitamin A (10,000 IU)
Zinc (15 milligrams)
Vitamin E (200 to 800 IU)
Selenium (200 to 300 micrograms)
L-cysteine (250 to 500 milligrams)
L-glutamine (250 to 1000 milligrams)

Nicotine Addiction

African Americans receive mixed messages. Public health officials warn of the dangers associated with cigarette smoking, while cigarette advertisers sell the public—*especially the African American public*—on the sex appeal and allure of smoking. While cigarette ads try to attract smokers of all races, African Americans have been the target of a concerted effort to recruit new addicts. In fact, recent court cases have forced the release of guarded industry documents demonstrating the importance of African American smokers in the tobacco market.

Despite the advertising claims, you already know that smoking is hazardous to your health, but you may not know the specifics: In the United States, smoking causes about 25 percent of all cancer deaths and 30 to 40 percent of deaths from heart disease. It also causes emphysema, peptic ulcers, and stroke, among other health problems. Take all of these factors into account, and you realize that cigarette smoking is the single most significant cause of preventable disease.

The nicotine in cigarettes makes them addictive; nicotine is a stimulant of the central nervous system and the cardiovascular system. A puff of smoke constricts blood vessels, which in turn increases blood pressure and forces the heart to work harder. The liver releases additional glycogen, raising the blood sugar. To the smoker, this state of cardiovascular stress, combined with a mild sugar rush, provides the "lift" or "up feeling" from smoking.

In addition to the nicotine, cigarette smoke contains at least four thousand chemicals, as well as tars and toxic gases, such as carbon monoxide, hydrogen cyanide, and nitrogen oxide. Cigarettes contain pesticides used to grow the tobacco and chemical additives used to keep the cigarette ablaze and to improve its taste. (If your cigarette does not extinguish itself when left alone, you can be certain that it has been chemically treated.) Other potentially deadly contaminants include arsenic, cyanide, lead, cadmium, dioxin (the most deadly pesticide known), and radioactive materials. (Someone who smokes 1½ packs of cigarettes a day is exposed to radiation equal to about three hundred chest X rays per year.)

Assuming this information has convinced you of the wisdom of kicking the habit, what can you do to strengthen your resolve and help you make it through withdrawal? First, switch to an alkaline diet high in raw fruits and vegetables. Increasing blood alkalinity helps reduce the craving for nicotine. A high-fiber, low-animal-fat diet can help keep your bowels moving smoothly during withdrawal. Taking up to five or six tablets of sodium or potassium bicarbonate throughout the day (during times of peak nicotine cravings) can help reduce acidity in the body during withdrawal. Continue with these dietary changes for at least four to six weeks.

(NOTE: If you have kidney problems, hypertension, or heart failure, consult your doctor before taking sodium or potassium supplements.)

Even with nutritional support, if you are addicted to nicotine, it won't be easy to quit. When we work with our patients who smoke, we first try to determine whether or not they are physically addicted to nicotine. People who are addicted to nicotine experience symptoms of withdrawal—nervousness, anger, sweating, and heart palpitations—if they go more than a couple of hours without a smoke. If you welcome the morning with a cigarette or put away more than two packs of cigarettes a day, chances are good you have a serious habit that will be a challenge to overcome—but you can do it.

Try to use the healing power of your mind by thinking about each cigarette before you light up. Ask yourself before smoking: "How am I feeling right now?" "Is there something else I can do for myself to pass the time until this craving passes?" Acknowledge your emotions and express them; this may help release the tension and help diminish the craving.

For some of our patients who are addicted, we may recommend using a nicotine patch that releases nicotine gradually into your system (available over the counter at drugstores). The patch approach can help smokers wean themselves off nicotine with reasonable success. The first day is the peak period of withdrawal and cravings may seem constant. Some smokers experience headaches, anxiety, dizziness, insomnia, and irritability as they work their way toward becoming ex-smokers. Other symptoms of withdrawal can include heart palpitations, inability to concentrate, depression, and stomach upset. You cannot smoke when wearing a nicotine patch without subjecting yourself to major health risks, including hypertension and heart problems.

Those people who have a cigarette habit rather than an addiction still have their work cut out for them. We try to get our patients to give up all but three or four cigarettes a day. In most cases, the last cigarettes to go are those they have with coffee and after meals. The attraction of these cigarettes is not the nicotine, but the familiarity of the habit.

With habitual smokers, we try to substitute one behavior for another. If the satisfaction associated with smoking seems to be oral, we might recommend that a patient try chewing gum or sucking a peppermint instead of smoking. If the satisfaction with these last cigarettes seems to focus on using the hands, we might suggest a patient try fiddling with a small toy or tying a string on a finger to keep the hands occupied. After we get down to the final four cigarettes, we have the patient give up one of those cigarettes a month.

Once you make up your mind to stop smoking, make a list of all the reasons you want to quit and read over the list at least once a day. Before you light up, think carefully about each cigarette and read over the list of reasons you want to quit. Then try waiting for ten or fifteen minutes, and if you still want the cigarette, you can have it. (The intense craving usually lasts less than five minutes.) While waiting, try one of your substitution acts to distract yourself.

If you feel anxious during withdrawal, consider using herbs to calm yourself. Tinctures of gotu kola, kava kava, and valerian can promote relaxation without the many negative side effects of smoking. We recommend looking for commercially prepared tinctures at health food stores; follow package directions. These treatments can be used for the four to six weeks of withdrawal as needed.

Reward yourself for each day you're smoke-free for the first week, then offer yourself incentives once a week after that. Every day—and every time you feel tempted to light up—remind yourself that you are now a nonsmoker. This will not only strengthen your resolve in the short term, it will also help change your self-image; over time you will internalize the message and you will in fact become a nonsmoker.

R̥ for Health

- Enroll in an antismoking program through the American Lung Association, the American Heart Association, or a local hospital. These programs usually combine education, exercise, and behavior modification.

- Acupuncture can help reduce nicotine cravings in some people. Contract a professional acupuncturist for support during the periods of withdrawal and detoxification.

- Experiment with herbs for relaxation. Tinctures of gotu kola, kava kava, and valerian can be particularly helpful; follow package directions. Use these herbs for four to six weeks.

- A number of supplemental antioxidants and other nutrients can reduce your cancer risk and protect your body during recovery. These supplements can be taken on an ongoing basis as a maintenance dose. Take the supplements for five of seven days of the week (weekends off). In addition to a good multiple vitamin/mineral supplement, take the following supplements:

Vitamin E (400 to 800 IU daily)
Selenium (200 to 300 micrograms daily)
Vitamin C (500 milligrams four or five times daily)
Coenzyme Q-10 (50 milligrams daily)
Copper (3 milligrams)
Zinc (15 milligrams daily)
L-cysteine (250 to 500 milligrams)

YOU'RE NOT IN THIS ALONE

Many people think they can work through their addictions on their own, but we have almost never seen this approach work. Addicts need to be held accountable—to themselves, to their medical practitioners (to keep appointments and be honest about what is going on in their lives), to other people (in a recovery group or a network that can offer much-needed support), and to their God or Higher Power (who can provide the strength and surrender required for spiritual growth).

Without appropriate support, many addicts can tough it out for a short period of time, but relapse is common and often the addict trades one addiction for another, alcohol for food or cigarettes, for example. In most cases, the addiction is a form of self-soothing, and the addict will seek out another habit or a cross addiction unless he or she gets healthy enough to heal the pain from within.

For more information on working through an addiction, consider contacting the following organizations:

Alcoholics Anonymous
(212) 870-3400 (or check the Yellow Pages for local listings)

American Lung Association
(800) 586-4872

Center for Substance Abuse Prevention
(800) 843-4971

Cocaine Anonymous
(800) COCAINE; (213) 559-5833

The Hazelden Foundation
(800) I-DO-CARE

Institute on Black Chemical Dependency
(612) 871-7878

Johnson Institute
(800) 231-5165; in Minnesota (800) 247-0484

Narcotics Anonymous
(800) 662-4357; (818) 780-3951

National Association of Alcoholism and Drug Abuse Counselors
(703) 920-4644

National Clearinghouse for Alcohol and Drug Information
(301) 468-2600

National Council on Alcoholism and Drug Dependence
(212) 206-6770

National Institute on Alcoholism and Drug Abuse
(800) 662-4357; (301) 443-4373

Office of Minority Health Resource Center
(800) 444-6472

Rational Recovery
(916) 621-4374

Secular Organizations for Sobriety (SOS)
(716) 834-2922

▼▼▼▼▼▼▼▼▼▼▼▼▼▼▼▼▼▼▼▼▼▼▼▼▼

ON THE SIDELINES

Most of us know someone who has an addiction problem. If the addict is someone close to us, we may think that we have the power to get the person to "change his ways," but we do not. It is up to the individual to choose the path of recovery; all we can do is stand on the sidelines and offer our love.

In order to support an addict, we may need to get support ourselves. We may, in fact, be helping them stay addicted, though this may not be our intention. No matter what, the person's addiction may be an opportunity for our healing. Your courage in healing may then be an example that can help the person you care about find the strength to move into recovery.

Support groups are very important because they can help you initiate change in yourself. The group needs to be loving, positive, and supportive. Find a group that supports those feelings in you and you will know that you have started on the journey of healing.

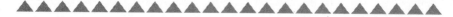

12

▼

Mending Our Hearts

Minimizing Your Risk of Cardiovascular Disease

Our African ancestors experienced very little cardiovascular disease. In fact, one fifteen-year study of 23,000 nomadic Africans in Ethiopia, Nigeria, and Kenya found absolutely *no* evidence of heart disease. One explanation for this extraordinary state of cardiovascular health may be the heart-healing benefits of the tribal diet, which is high in vegetables and grains and low in fat (about 10 percent of calories come from fat). Perhaps because of this healthy diet, the average cholesterol level of the Africans in the study was a low 131, compared with the American average cholesterol level of 210 to 220.

By getting back to our roots and sharing in a similar healthy lifestyle and diet plan, most of us can enjoy improved cardiovascular health—and we may even be able to reverse early stages of cardiovascular disease. We have seen dramatic results among our patients who switch to a heart-smart way of life. For example, a few years ago a thirty-six-year-old woman came to us for help controlling her hypertension. She was twenty-five pounds overweight and her blood pressure was 140/92 despite the fact that she was taking three different antihypertensive drugs prescribed by another doctor. We put her on a low-carbohydrate diet, recommended that she walk fifteen minutes three times a week,

213

and gave her a series of nutritional supplements, including garlic, magnesium, calcium, fish oil, and taurine.

Within one month, her blood pressure had dropped to 118/80 and she had lost seven pounds. We weaned her from the prescription medications, and over the next two months she lost eleven pounds more and her blood pressure fell to 118/76. Three months after walking into our office, this woman looked five years younger. She had also normalized her blood pressure, lost weight, and regained her energy—all using nothing but natural treatments.

Heart disease and hypertension do require careful monitoring by a physician, but we have found that these conditions respond very well to natural treatments. The body is willing to heal itself if given the chance. Sometimes natural methods work, even when the patient proves less than cooperative. Consider the sixty-two-year-old African American smoker who came to us with severe circulation problems in his legs due to hardening of the arteries. His calves cramped, the hair on his legs fell out, and he developed black blisters on his toes—early signs of gangrene. He steadfastly refused to allow a surgeon to open up the arteries in his legs, and instead came to us for treatment using natural medicine. Though skeptical of the likelihood of success considering the severity of his symptoms, we prescribed two Chinese herbal formulations designed to improve circulation. Within two weeks, the blisters vanished, the leg cramps disappeared, and the man could walk farther than he had been able to for years. For the past two years, he has experienced no relapse, despite his stubborn refusal to quit smoking.

Taking steps to improve our cardiovascular health is particularly important for African Americans. Heart disease is the number one killer of Americans of all races, but the problem is greatest among African Americans, probably because we suffer disproportionately from high blood pressure. A 1987 study found that the rate of heart disease was 27 percent greater in black men than in white men, and a remarkable 55 percent greater in black women than in white women. In order to improve our overall health, we must improve our cardiovascular health.

MATTERS OF THE HEART: UNDERSTANDING HEART DISEASE

Each day, your heart beats about 100,000 times, pumping blood through the body's 12,400-mile network of arteries, veins, and blood vessels. This complex system circulates life-giving oxygen throughout the body, nourishing every cell. When any part of the system fails, the entire body is put at risk; cardiovascular disease claims about one million lives each year. Following is a brief description of the most common forms of cardiovascular disease:

- HEART ATTACK. The heart is a muscle. If it is deprived of oxygen, all or part of the muscle dies; this is what we refer to as a heart attack (or myocardial infarction). Each year, more than 1.5 million Americans suffer heart attacks and about one out of three of them dies.

    Blood clots cause many heart attacks; when blood flows through an artery that has been narrowed by atherosclerosis, it slows down and tends to clot. When the clot becomes big enough, it completely blocks the flow of blood, causing a heart attack. An irregular heartbeat (or arrhythmia) can also cause heart attack if it is severe enough to prevent enough blood from reaching the heart muscle.

▼▼▼▼▼▼▼▼▼▼▼▼▼▼▼▼▼▼▼▼▼▼▼▼▼

ARE YOU HAVING A HEART ATTACK?

Heart attack victims often delay seeking medical help—sometimes with fatal results. Most heart attack deaths occur in the first two hours, yet studies have found that many people wait four to six hours to get to an emergency room when they think they may be having a heart attack. We urge our patients to contact us immediately if they experience any cardiac warning signs. Never ignore the warning signs of heart attack, which include:

- Chest pain. An uncomfortable pressure, fullness, squeezing, or crushing feeling in the center of the chest that lasts two minutes or longer

- Severe pain that radiates to the shoulders, neck, arms, jaw, or top of the stomach

- Paleness

- Sweating

- Rapid or irregular pulse

- Dizziness, fainting, or loss of consciousness

Not all of these warning signs occur with every heart attack. And some people, especially African Americans, may not experience symptoms during a heart attack. (These so-called silent heart attacks can be detected only by an electrocardiogram.) If you suspect you may be experiencing a heart attack, seek emergency help immediately. Doctors can prescribe a number of drugs that dissolve clots and reduce the oxygen demands of the heart, but these medications are most effective if given within one hour of the onset of a heart attack. Time is of the essence.

- ANGINA. When the heart muscle is starved for oxygen (but receives enough to stay alive), the result can be an excruciating episode of angina pectoris. In most cases, the pain starts with constriction in the center of the chest, then radiates to the throat, back, neck, jaw, and down the left arm; it is usually accompanied by breathlessness, nausea, and dizziness. Most attacks last five minutes or so and occur when the heart, damaged by high blood pressure and coronary artery disease, is stressed by physical exertion, emotional upset, excessive excitement, or even digestion of a heavy meal.

- ATHEROSCLEROSIS. Hardening of the arteries, or atherosclerosis, involves the buildup of fatty deposits or plaque in the arteries. The deposits narrow the arteries, reducing the blood supply to the heart and increasing the likelihood of a blood clot clogging an arterial pathway and causing a heart attack.

  In most cases, atherosclerosis occurs after the arteries develop tiny tears (often caused by the powerful pumping of the heart in someone with high blood pressure). Sludgy cholesterol in the blood then accumulates in the tears, gradually hardening and forming plaque. These plaque deposits then narrow the passageways, cutting down the blood supply.

Because the circulatory system is so efficient, many people develop severe cardiovascular disease before any symptoms appear. In fact, the vessels can be 70 to 90 percent blocked before signs of illness appear. Unfortunately, a heart attack is often the first warning sign that something is wrong.

- CONGESTIVE HEART FAILURE. When the heart muscle has been damaged to the point that it can no longer pump efficiently, the result is congestive heart failure. When the heart grows weak, the kidneys respond to the reduced blood circulation by retaining salt and water in the body, which further stresses the heart and makes the situation worse.

  Congestive heart failure can occur on either the right or left side of the heart. The left side of the heart pumps oxygen-rich blood from the lungs to the rest of the body; when this part of the heart is damaged, blood backs up in the lungs, resulting in wheezing, shortness of breath, fatigue, sleep problems, and a dry, hacking, nonproductive cough (especially when lying down). The right side of the heart pumps the oxygen-depleted blood from the body to the lungs; when this part of the heart is damaged, the blood collects in the legs and liver, causing swollen feet, ankles, and neck veins, as well as lethargy and pain below the ribs.

- STROKE. Just as a heart attack involves oxygen deprivation of the heart, a stroke involves oxygen deprivation of the brain. There are several types of stroke: A thrombotic stroke occurs when an artery in the brain is blocked by a clot or atherosclerosis; an embolic stroke occurs when a small clot (known as an embolus) forms elsewhere in the body and moves to the brain, where it lodges in an artery and blocks the flow of blood; and a hemorrhagic stroke occurs when an artery ruptures, usually due to high blood pressure. Hemorrhagic strokes tend to be most deadly; they account for about 20 percent of all strokes but 50 percent of all stroke-related deaths.

  During a stroke, part of the brain dies due to a lack of oxygen.

In fact, strokes are the leading cause of adult disability. Symptoms of a stroke include slurred speech or loss of speech, sudden severe headache, double vision or blindness, sudden weakness or loss of sensation in the limbs, or loss of consciousness. These symptoms can occur over a period of a few minutes or hours, and they can occur on one side of the body or both. Stroke is the third leading cause of death in African Americans; it is estimated that the mortality rate from strokes among African Americans is approximately 66 percent higher than among whites, probably due to our high levels of hypertension.

THE LOWDOWN ON HIGH BLOOD PRESSURE

Hypertension (or high blood pressure) is a leading health problem among blacks. In the United States, some sixty million people suffer from hypertension—and an astounding one out of every three of them is black. In fact, hypertension is twice as common in blacks as whites, and severe hypertension is five times more common in black men and seven times more common in black women compared with whites. Blacks develop hypertension earlier than whites and tend to suffer its worst consequences.

Hypertension is more than a medical annoyance; it is the most accurate predictor of future cardiovascular disease in people above age sixty-five. At the most basic level, hypertension refers to the pressure of the blood against the blood vessels as the heart pumps the blood through the arteries. A blood pressure reading consists of two numbers: the systolic pressure (the higher number, reflecting the pressure when the heart contracts) and the diastolic pressure (the lower number, reflecting the pressure as the heart rests between beats).

A normal blood pressure reading is 120/80, though the numbers fluctuate somewhat throughout the day. If your blood pressure is 140/90 or higher, you have hypertension and need to work on lowering it. We believe that hypertension cannot be cured, but it can—and must—be controlled. Untreated, high blood pressure can lead to stroke, heart disease and heart attack, loss of vision, and kidney failure because the heart must work harder than normal to pump blood. In fact, people with hypertension face a risk of heart attack three times greater and a risk of stroke seven times greater than that of people with normal blood pressure.

For a number of reasons, African Americans suffer disproportionately from hypertension. As far back as 1932, researchers found clear differences in blood pressure rates between blacks and whites of all ages, though the major differences tend to show up after age seventeen.

One theory to explain the high rate of hypertension is that blacks have inherited an unusual response to the intake of salt. According to this unproven hypothesis, most people excrete excess sodium through their sweat and urine, but many blacks retain sodium in their kidneys. The retained sodium helps the body conserve fluids, which may have been a genetic advantage in the arid African climate, but in today's world, fluid retention can strain the heart and lead to high blood pressure. About 75 percent of blacks with hypertension are salt sensitive, twice the rate of whites.

Hypertension is often called "the silent killer" because it strikes without warning. Advanced hypertension can sometimes cause headache (especially in the morning), fatigue, dizziness, rapid pulse, shortness of breath, sweating, nosebleeds, and visual problems. The only way to be sure your blood pressure is under control is to have it checked; you can either get a home monitor and learn how to use it, or visit your doctor regularly and have your blood pressure checked. Fortunately, most cases of high blood pressure can be lowered by making lifestyle adjustments and following the general advice for strengthening the cardiovascular system. Some cases require prescription medication, but a healthy lifestyle and the use of natural supplements can dramatically reduce the need for drugs in most people.

▼▼▼▼▼▼▼▼▼▼▼▼▼▼▼▼▼▼▼▼▼▼▼▼▼

HOW HIGH IS HIGH?

Stage 1 hypertension: Systolic pressure of 140 to 159
                             Diastolic pressure of 90 to 99

Stage 2 hypertension: Systolic pressure of 160 to 179
           Diastolic pressure of 100 to 109
Stage 3 hypertension: Systolic pressure of 180 to 209
           Diastolic pressure of 110 to 119
Stage 4 hypertension: Systolic pressure of 210 or more
           Diastolic pressure of 120 or more

▲▲▲▲▲▲▲▲▲▲▲▲▲▲▲▲▲▲▲▲▲▲▲▲▲▲▲▲

OPENING YOUR HEART: SPIRITUALITY AND HEART DISEASE

Spiritually, the heart is the source of our loving and the center of our emotions. Physically, the heart is the source of our pulse and the central pump of our circulatory system. For the heart and circulatory system to function their best, both the spirit and body must be free of tension and emotional turmoil. In many cases, cardiovascular disease is a physical manifestation of emotional conflict and stress.

When our patients come to us with concern about their cardiovascular health, they often tell us, "Heart disease runs in my family." These people are referring to their genetic inheritance, but we explain to them that their risk of heart disease goes beyond their genetic makeup. In addition to the physical propensity toward illness (or wellness) that we inherit from our parents, we also receive an emotional inheritance; we learn from our parents (and other family members) how to handle and express our emotions. Families that tend to suppress emotions or to express their emotions with hostility or in other inappropriate ways create stress and emotional conflicts that can actually contribute to cardiovascular disease. In many cases, this emotional legacy can be as important a cardiovascular disease risk factor as a family history of heart disease.

As we have seen time and again with our patients, heart disease can be significantly improved in many cases by learning to accept and express our emotions. To heal the heart, we recommend "emotional open-heart surgery" for all our patients. In other words, we urge our patients to open their hearts to their emotional truth. In many cases, people try to suppress the emotions that make them feel uncomfortable, but it is impossible to suppress one emotion without suppressing all emotions, including love. Emotional, spiritual, and physical health depend on your ability to open your heart fully.

To open your heart, you must learn to speak your emotional truth; you must learn to allow yourself to experience what you are feeling right now. When we ask our patients how they are feeling, quite often we are told, "I don't know." This is not an acceptable response; "I don't know" is a convenient excuse for keeping your emotions buried. Instead of hiding, you must learn to look beneath "I don't know" and to discover the emotions that you are trying to dismiss. This suppression of emotion results in tension and stress that will over time contribute to cardiovascular disease. (For more information on managing your emotions, see Chapter 4, "Attitude Is Everything," page 59.)

The physical expression of love—making love—also helps to heal the heart. During intercourse and orgasm, blood rushes to the peripheral organs, and the tissues of the body (including the arteries) relax. So a vital sex life with a loving partner may strengthen your heart both emotionally and physically.

The love of a pet also helps relieve stress and improve cardiovascular health. Pets offer unconditional love, and they depend on us for their food and shelter. A number of studies have shown the health benefits of loving an animal. For example, one study of elderly people in a nursing home found that those who had a chance to snuggle and stroke a pet two or three times a week experienced lower blood pressure both during the time they interacted with the animal and for hours afterward.

The emotional components of cardiovascular health have become more widely accepted in recent years, in part due to the demonstrated success of Dr. Dean Ornish's program for reversing cardiovascular disease. In addition to moderate exercise and an ultra-low-fat diet, his program includes meditation, Yoga, and group support. Our experiences with our patients resemble those of Dr. Ornish: To control heart disease, diet alone is not enough; exercise alone is not enough. You must also open your heart to yourself and those you love.

UNDERSTANDING CHOLESTEROL

Study after study has shown that the higher your level of blood cholesterol, the greater your chances of dying from heart disease. A total blood cholesterol level of 240 or greater doubles your risk of heart disease. But we remind our patients—especially those with elevated cholesterol levels—that the reverse is also true: For every 1 percent you lower your total cholesterol level, you reduce your heart disease risk by 2 to 3 percent.

To assess your cardiovascular risk profile, you need to determine your total cholesterol level. In general, the lower the number, the better. A total cholesterol level below 180 milligrams/deciliter is ideal, but you must also consider the type of cholesterol.

Before the cholesterol can enter the bloodstream it must attach itself to a molecule known as a lipoprotein. (Cholesterol is a fatlike substance, and blood is essentially water; the lipoprotein helps to transport the cholesterol through the blood because fat and water don't mix.) There are two main types of lipoproteins—low-density lipoproteins (LDLs) and high-density lipoproteins (HDLs). LDLs contribute to the formation of plaque deposits in the arteries and HDLs help to remove those plaque deposits from the arteries. When a person has high LDL and low HDL levels, the blood often contains high levels of triglycerides (another blood fat) as well. High triglyceride levels are common in diabetics and people who are obese.

Cardiovascular disease can be caused by either too little HDL or too much LDL. To minimize your risk of cardiovascular disease, you should aim for low levels of LDL cholesterol and high levels of HDL cholesterol. You can raise your HDLs by exercising and eating a diet rich in fruits and vegetables, as well as by not smoking and by avoiding saturated fats. You can lower your LDL level by avoiding saturated fats and sugars, and by eating sufficient amounts of vitamin C and chromium. We recommend limiting your cholesterol intake to about 300 milligrams per day (the amount in one egg yolk). The average daily intake in the United States is 500 milligrams for men and 350 milligrams for women.

Though cholesterol has earned a bad reputation for clogging the arteries, it is actually essential for a number of bodily processes, including nerve function, reproduction, hormone production, and the formation of cell membranes. While cholesterol is found in some of the foods we eat, most of it is manufactured by the liver. In fact, each day our bodies churn out about 1000 milligrams of the waxy white stuff.

Your Target Cholesterol Level

	Desirable	Borderline	Undesirable
Total cholesterol	below 200	200–239	240+
LDL cholesterol	below 130	130–159	160+
HDL cholesterol	above 45	35–45	below 35

There is more to the story than your total cholesterol level. In assessing the risk of cardiovascular disease, we focus more on the ratio of HDL to total cholesterol levels. (To find this number, take the total cholesterol level and divide by the HDL level. For example, if your total cholesterol were 200 and your HDL were 50, your ratio would be 4.) We like to see our patients with a ratio of 4 or less.

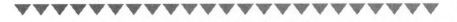

THE HOMOCYSTEINE CONNECTION

You can control some cardiovascular disease risk factors; others you can't. One significant risk factor that you can eliminate with a simple vitamin supplement is your homocysteine level.

Homocysteine is an amino acid that can damage the cardiovascular system when it is present at high levels. Diets deficient in vitamin B_6, vitamin B_{12}, or folate can lead to dangerously high blood levels of homocysteine, contributing to heart disease.

Roughly one out of every eight people inherits a gene that increases the likelihood of homocysteine buildup by slowing the body's disposal of the substance. Patterns of homocysteine levels also track with incidence of heart disease. For example, women's homocysteine levels are about 20 percent below men's during their reproductive years, but their homocysteine levels (and risk of heart disease) increase after menopause. In addition, homocysteine levels and incidence of cardiovascular disease increase with age, as the body becomes less adept at absorbing B vitamins.

Fortunately, the problem can be resolved by eating a diet containing a sufficient amount of the B vitamins, or by taking a B vitamin supplement. We encourage our patients to take supplemental B vitamins; in many cases we also recommend a simple blood test to measure homocysteine levels. (The test usually costs $50 to $120, and it may be covered by your health insurance company.)

▲▲▲▲▲▲▲▲▲▲▲▲▲▲▲▲▲▲▲▲▲▲▲▲▲▲

HEART-SMART APPROACH TO HEALTHY LIVING

While not all cardiovascular disease depends on lifestyle, there are many things you can do to keep your heart and circulatory system in top shape. We recommend the following:

- **Exercise.** A healthy heart is an exercised heart. Aerobic exercise helps prevent cardiovascular disease by lowering LDL cholesterol levels and raising HDL cholesterol levels, reducing blood pressure, keeping weight down, burning fat, lowering blood sugar levels, and promoting relaxation. People who exercise regularly are about half as likely as sedentary people to have a heart attack. In addition, studies have found that people who exercised as part of their rehabilitation after a heart attack had a 25-percent reduction in second heart attacks. See Chapter 8, "Working It Out," page 127, for more information on exercise and aerobic conditioning.

- **Learn stress management.** You need to become aware of your anger, anxiety, and fear. Negative emotions trigger the release of adrenaline and increase blood pressure. These hormones also encourage the cells to release fat and cholesterol into the bloodstream. For information on stress management, see the recommendations in Chapter 4, "Attitude Is Everything," page 59. We also recommend that people read *The Relaxation Response* by Herbert Benson.

- **Don't smoke.** Smokers have two to four times the risk of having a heart attack as nonsmokers, and their heart attacks are more likely to be fatal. Nicotine constricts arteries, elevates blood pressure, speeds atherosclerosis, and reduces oxygen levels in the blood.

While there has been a nationwide decline in the rate of smoking in the United States, the decline is less among blacks, especially young black women. A person with uncontrolled hypertension who smokes is five times more likely to have a heart attack and sixteen times more likely to have a stroke than a nonsmoker. Now a bit of good news: A decade after quitting, a former pack-a-day smoker has almost the same heart attack risk as if he had never smoked.

- **Maintain healthy weight.** Being 20 percent or more above your desirable weight doubles your risk of developing heart disease. Those extra pounds raise blood pressure, increase total cholesterol levels, and reduce levels of "good" HDL cholesterol. For more information on weight control, see Chapter 7, "Reshaping Your Body," page 115.

- **Eat a high-fiber diet.** A high-fiber diet helps lower cholesterol levels. The average American consumes only 11 grams of fiber a day, far short of the 25 grams we recommend. Strive to obtain as much fiber as possible from the foods you eat. However, if you don't care for high-fiber foods or don't eat enough of them, take a psyllium-based supplement (follow package directions). One study found that people who took one tablespoon of soluble-fiber supplement twice a day for eight weeks had a 7-percent reduction in their LDL cholesterol levels. (Fiber tablets won't provide the same cholesterol-lowering benefits since they contain a synthetic, insoluble form of fiber.)

- **Limit your use of alcohol.** While some researchers tout the cardiovascular benefits of modest drinking, consuming more than 30 ml of alcohol a day—an amount equal to one ounce of 100-proof whiskey, eight ounces of wine, or two 12-ounce beers—can raise blood pressure.

- **Restrict your sodium intake.** The sodium in salt (sodium chloride) makes the body retain fluids, which in turn raises blood pressure and forces your heart to work harder. Read all food labels carefully, keeping an eye out for foods containing soda, sodium, or the symbol "Na" on the label. In addition, avoid high-sodium foods such as smoked or aged cheeses and meats, chocolate, animal fats, gravy, bouillon, and processed foods.

R̳ for Health

In addition to working with your regular doctor or health care professional to manage any cardiovascular problems you might have, consider using natural remedies to improve your cardiovascular health. The following supplements can be taken as a maintenance dose on an ongoing basis. Take them five days a week, with weekends off.

- **Take 3 to 10 garlic cloves daily.** Garlic is a powerful blood pressure–lowering agent; it also thins the blood and reduces triglycerides, cholesterol, and LDL, while raising HDL. Consume 3 to 10 cloves of fresh garlic a day, or use commercial garlic preparations, following package directions. You can use odorless garlic since the cardiovascular benefits have nothing to do with the garlic's being fresh.

  NOTE: According to Paul Yanick, Ph.D., in some people, garlic can create a bile duct spasm that blocks the liver detoxification pathways. If you experience constipation or dizziness when you take garlic, consult your doctor or health care provider. Garlic can also create energetic symptoms (such as ringing in the ears and hot flashes), which will subside when you stop taking garlic.

- **Take 50 milligrams of B_6, 50 milligrams of B_{12}, and 400 micrograms of folate a day.** These B vitamins help to lower homocysteine levels in the blood, reducing the risk of developing cardiovascular disease.

- **Take 400 to 800 IU of vitamin E and 1 gram of vitamin C daily.** These antioxidants help prevent free radical damage, in addition to helping the body maintain the heart muscle. Vitamin E helps prevent LDL cholesterol from oxidizing and forming plaque deposits in the arteries. Several studies have shown that the lower the levels of vitamin C in a person's bloodstream, the higher that person's blood pressure. One study found that taking as little as 250 milligrams of vitamin C a day slashed the risk of high blood pressure by almost half. Vitamin C is essential for the excretion of excess cholesterol from the body, and it helps the body balance HDL and LDL cholesterol.

- **Eat 20 to 25 grams of soy two to three times a week.** This protein contains two phytoestrogens—genistein and deidzen—that appear to help clear cholesterol from the blood. An analysis of thirty-eight clinical trials found that people who ate an average of 47 grams of soy daily had a 13-percent drop in harmful LDL cholesterol levels and a 9-percent drop in their total cholesterol level. (The soy did not affect the level of helpful HDL cholesterol.) You can consume 20 to 25 grams of soy by eating 5 or 6 ounces of tofu.

▼▼▼▼▼▼▼▼▼▼▼▼▼▼▼▼▼▼▼▼▼▼▼▼

Other Supplements to Consider

In addition to the primary supplements listed above, we also recommend taking one or more of the following supplements during times of emotional or physical stress. You can take these additional supplements for up to four weeks.

- **Calcium (250 milligrams) and magnesium (500 milligrams) daily.** Calcium is essential for blood clotting; it also plays a role in maintaining blood pressure. Magnesium is necessary to normalize the heartbeat. It activates an enzyme that helps transport potassium to the cells, so if the body is deficient in magnesium, the potassium balance is disturbed and arrthymias may result. Many African Americans do not consume enough magnesium in their diet. Magnesium also helps keep calcium in circulation so that it does not precipitate in tissues, a significant factor in atherosclerosis.

- **Fish oil (1 gram) three times a day.** Fish oil lowers blood pressure and thins the blood. Also include fish in your diet at least two or three times per week.

- **Taurine (200 milligrams) daily.** Taurine is an amino acid found in high concentrations in the heart, central nervous system, and white blood cells. It helps stabilize the heartbeat by correcting cardiac arrhythmias.

- **Carnitine (900 milligrams) twice a day.** This vitamin-like compound helps the heart use oxygen more efficiently. In the body, carnitine assists in the transportation and breakdown of fatty acids in the cells.

- **Coenzyme Q-10 (30 to 50 milligrams) daily.** In the heart, coenzyme Q-10 helps prevent the accumulation of fatty acids; it also plays a critical role in energy production in the cells. It has been shown to increase heart contractions and to smooth out some abnormal heart rhythms.

Three Herbs for Your Heart

While a number of herbs can be used to strengthen the heart and control cardiovascular disease, we have had the most luck with these three. Consider adding these herbs to your supplements during periods of stress and for one week during the change of seasons:

- **Hawthorn.** This so-called heart herb enhances cardiac output, opens up the peripheral vessels to improve overall circulation, and prevents cholesterol deposit from forming on artery walls. For an infusion, use 2 teaspoons of crushed leaves per cup of boiling water. Steep 20 minutes, strain, and drink up to 2 cups a day. Commercially prepared tinctures are also available; follow package directions.

- **Yarrow.** This herb improves blood flow and lowers blood pressure by relaxing the peripheral blood vessels and working as a diuretic. Commercially prepared tinctures are available from health food stores; follow the package directions.

- **Celery.** Eating celery (as well as consuming celery oil and ground celery seeds) helps to lower blood pressure by relaxing the smooth muscles in the blood vessels. Chomping on as few as four stalks of celery a day provides enough of the active ingredient, a compound known as 3-butylphthalide, to reduce blood pressure.

▲▲▲▲▲▲▲▲▲▲▲▲▲▲▲▲▲▲▲▲▲▲▲▲▲▲▲▲

▼▼▼▼▼▼▼▼▼▼▼▼▼▼▼▼▼▼▼▼▼▼▼▼▼▼

ACUPRESSURE FOR A HEALTHY HEART

Acupressure can be helpful in calming and strengthening the heart. To bolster your circulatory system and stimulate your heart, use one or more of the acupressure points listed below. Acupressure can be practiced on an ongoing basis. (For more information on the use of acupressure and diagrams of the points, see Chapter 2, "East Meets West," page 13.)

- *Bladder 15.* This point is located two finger widths outside either side of the spine, approximately halfway between the shoulder blades. This point relieves heart palpitations and improves overall heart function.

- *Conception Vessel 17.* Place your fingers along the midline of your chest in line with the nipples. This is the most tender spot along the breastbone. This point helps relieve heart palpitations; it also improves heart and lung function.

- *Heart 3.* This point is located on the inside of the elbow at the inside edge of the crease when the elbow is flexed. This point relieves cardiac pain and constriction in the chest.

- *Heart 7.* With your palm facing upward, this point is located on the outside edge of the wrist crease closest to the palm, in the hollow level with the little finger. This point improves circulation and strengthens the heart.

- *Pericardium 4.* Place your fingers on the inside of the forearm, halfway between the wrist and the elbow, in line with the middle finger, in the depression between the tendons. This point relieves cardiac pain and heart palpitations.

- *Pericardium 6.* This point is located three finger widths above the wrist crease closest to the palm, between the tendons on the inside of the arm. This point relieves chest pain associated with angina, stimulates heart function, and promotes good circulation, especially in the arms and chest.

- *Stomach 36.* Place your fingers four finger widths below the kneecap on the outside edge of the leg bone. This point improves overall circulation.

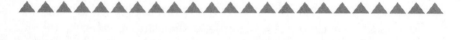

Dr. Singleton on Chelation Therapy

I have had a lot of success treating patients with chelation therapy. This treatment involves the intravenous infusion of a prescription medicine into the bloodstream to clean plaque from the arteries.

Though it sounds complex, the process is actually quite simple. The medicine—a combination of vitamins, minerals, and EDTA (ethylene-diamine tetra-acetic acid)—binds with calcium, as well as lead, mercury, cadmium, and other heavy metals, and removes them from the blood. Once the calcium and heavy metals have been flushed from the cells, the plaque deposits shrink and the blood vessels become more supple and healthier.

Chelation therapy isn't new; the U.S. Food and Drug Administration approved it for the treatment of lead poisoning more than thirty years ago. (It has not, however, been formally approved for the treatment of cardiovascular disease.) Conservative physicians argue that chelation therapy hasn't been adequately tested. I have researched the question, and I administered the treatment to myself before giving it to any of my patients. After the treatment, I felt thoroughly detoxified; many of my patients have reported an improvement in heart pain, as well as notable improvements in their hearing, vision, and memory. Some also said the treatment helped to normalize their irregular heartbeat.

Like any other treatment, chelation therapy is not for everyone. People with kidney problems should not try it (the drug is excreted through the urine). In addition, the side effects can include fever, headache, and fatigue. However, when you weigh the risks and benefits of the treatment, it makes sense for many patients.

FOR MORE INFORMATION

American Heart Association
7272 Greenville Ave.
Dallas, TX 75231
214-373-6300

International Atherosclerosis Society
6550 Fannin, No. 1423
Houston, TX 77030
713-790-4226

National Heart, Lung, and Blood Institute
Information Center
National Institutes of Health
301-251-1222

National Hypertension Association
324 E. 30th St.
New York, NY 10016
212-889-3557

American Society of Hypertension
515 Madison Ave., Suite 1212
New York, NY 10022
212-644-0650

**Citizens for Public Action on Blood Pressure
and Cholesterol**
P.O. Box 30374
Bethesda, MD 20824
301-770-1711

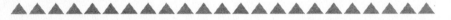

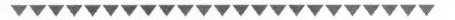

OUR HERITAGE OF HEALING

In the tropical countries of Africa, our ancestors often ate okro, or "ladyfingers," a heart-healing vegetable that is known as okra in the United States. Okra *(Hibiscus esculentus)* provides the protective and healing nutrients found in many dark green vegetables, but it also contains a unique mucilage or soluble fiber that helps lower blood cholesterol levels.

Spiced Okra
Serves 4

Okra is used in Africa and in the United States in soups, stews, and side dishes. If you cook okra quickly, it will remain firm; slower cooking will result in the traditional softer, more gelatinous texture.

¼ cup minced onion
1 small garlic clove, minced
¼ teaspoon cayenne
Salt and black pepper
⅓ pound fresh okra, cut into 1-inch-long pieces

Combine 1 cup of water, the onion, garlic, cayenne, and salt and black pepper to taste in a saucepan. Bring to a boil. Add the okra and cook about 15 minutes, until almost all the liquid is absorbed. Drain the okra in a colander and run cold water over it to stop the cooking. Chill before serving and enjoy.

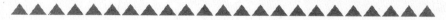

13

▼

Avoiding the Highs and Lows

Stabilizing Our Blood Sugar Levels

Diabetes is a quiet killer. It is the third leading cause of death among African Americans, but at least half of the people who suffer from the condition don't know they are sick. Compared to whites, African Americans suffer from diabetes twice as often; we also develop it at younger ages and experience higher rates of the most serious complications, including cardiovascular disease, blindness, amputation, and kidney failure.

Before the turn of the century, diabetes was almost unheard of among African Americans. But today blacks have higher rates of diabetes than whites at all age levels, primarily due to the changes in our diet. African Americans (as well as Native Americans and Hawaiians) began developing diabetes in large numbers when we began eating a highly processed, high-animal-fat Western diet. In essence, the foods we began to eat no longer matched the genetic demands of what we should eat.

Our vulnerability to this disease begins early and increases as we grow older. Between the ages of forty-five and sixty-five, one out of ten African Americans suffers from diabetes, twice the rate of whites of the same age. Over the age of sixty-five, we have almost three times the incidence. The disease afflicts an astonishing number of older African American women: Over the age of fifty-five, one out of four has diabetes. In general, our susceptibility to diabetes reflects the change in our eating patterns, trace mineral deficiencies, and the increased use of foods that increase inflammation in our bodies.

For diabetics, life is a balancing act. Their bodies do not properly make or use insulin, so they must carefully watch their blood sugar numbers: If blood sugar levels rise too high for too long, they risk damage to the nerves and blood vessels, which can cause a number of health problems, including blindness, infections, kidney problems, stroke, and heart disease. But if blood sugar levels drop too low—even for a few minutes—they can become confused and even lose consciousness.

Normally, the pancreas regulates this delicate balance of sugar in the bloodstream. But the fourteen million Americans with diabetes mellitus cannot properly convert food, especially sugar, into energy, either because their bodies do not produce enough insulin (a hormone produced in the pancreas to regulate blood sugar levels) or because their bodies don't properly use the insulin they do produce. Instead, diabetics must monitor their blood sugar levels, adjusting their diet and exercise—or their oral medications and insulin injections—to meet these changing conditions. In addition, they should strive to reduce the stress on the pancreas through changes in diet and the use of nutritional supplements.

There are two basic types of diabetes: the more severe form, known as Type I, insulin-dependent, or juvenile diabetes (about 15 percent of cases), and Type II, non-insulin-dependent, or adult-onset diabetes (about 85 percent of cases).

- Type I diabetes usually strikes sometime between the onset of puberty and age thirty. It is caused by damage to the insulin-producing cells in the pancreas. For some reason, it affects males more often than females. The symptoms of Type I diabetes—excessive thirst, frequent urination, dry mouth, extreme hunger, weight loss, weakness, nausea, blurred vision, and frequent infections—often develop rapidly.

- Type II diabetes usually occurs in middle-aged and older people, especially those who are overweight. With Type II diabetes, the pancreas produces insulin, but the sugar remains in the blood-

stream. This more subtle version of the disease often goes undetected until complications arise. The signs of Type II diabetes—
thirst, drowsiness, obesity, fatigue, tingling or numbness in the feet,
blurred vision, urinary tract infections, slow healing of cuts, and
itching—often go unrecognized for years before being properly
diagnosed. Ultimately, up to 60 percent of Type II diabetics need
supplemental insulin. Obesity is a major contributing factor to Type
II diabetes. Among people with diagnosed diabetes, 82 percent of
adult black women are obese and 45 percent of black men are
obese. Losing as little as ten to fifteen pounds helps control Type II
diabetes in most cases.

Both Type I and Type II diabetes seem to have a genetic component as well. Another possible cause is an immune response following a
viral infection, which destroys the cells in the pancreas. Diabetes can
also follow other diseases, such as thyroid disorders, inflammation of
the pancreas, or problems with the pituitary gland. In addition, about 5
percent of women develop diabetes when pregnant, though the symptoms usually disappear after the baby is born.

Fortunately, Type II diabetes can often be prevented and responds
very well to natural treatments. The treatments we recommend in this
chapter can help you manage diabetes, but you should be under the
care of a physician or other medical professional if you have been diagnosed with the disease.

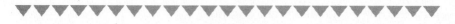

Is It Diabetes?

If you are overweight, over forty, or have a family history of diabetes, you might want to encourage your physician to test for diabetes at your annual physical. According to the U.S. National
Institutes of Health, you may be diabetic if your blood glucose level
is equal to or greater than 125 milligrams per deciliter of blood first
thing in the morning, if your blood glucose level is equal to or
greater than 200 mg/dl two hours after consuming 75 grams of

glucose, or if you experience hyperglycemia (a random glucose level of more than 200 mg/dl). A simple blood test for glucose levels can be performed at a doctor's office.

▲▲▲▲▲▲▲▲▲▲▲▲▲▲▲▲▲▲▲▲▲▲▲▲▲▲▲▲▲

LIVING WITH DIABETES

The standard treatment for diabetes focuses on controlling blood sugar levels, relieving symptoms, and preventing complications associated with the disease. To confirm the diagnosis, a doctor can administer a glucose tolerance test, which measures the body's reaction to sugar. Maintaining a healthy weight through a balanced diet and exercise is the single most important thing you can do to prevent and manage diabetes. In some cases, medication and insulin injections may be needed to lower blood sugar levels.

Diabetics must also take steps to protect their feet, teeth, and gums. Nerve damage associated with the disease can reduce sensation in the feet, leaving them susceptible to injuries and infections, which don't heal well due to blood vessel damage. Simple cuts and scrapes can easily become gangrenous. In addition, diabetics tend to develop more tooth and gum infections.

While you should never stop taking insulin or adjust your medication without consulting your doctor, many natural treatments can be very effective in handling the condition.

• TREATING TYPE I. There isn't much you can do to prevent Type I diabetes, but there are steps you can take to protect your nerves, eyes, and kidneys from damage caused by high blood sugar levels. If we see a person with Type I diabetes in the first few months of the disease, we give them niacinamide (a variant of the B vitamin niacin) to prevent further damage to the pancreas. We also have the patient avoid milk and dairy products because we believe there is an autoimmune component with some Type I diabetics related to milk proteins. In our experience, eliminating milk from the diet can help lower insulin requirements, and it minimizes cell loss in the pancreas.

- TREATING TYPE II. Adult-onset diabetes involves a more complex metabolic process, linked to obesity and diet. Type II diabetes is potentially curable (some people will need lifelong treatment because their pancreas was damaged before the diabetes was recognized and managed). In most cases, Type II diabetes can be controlled through diet, weight control, and exercise without taking supplemental insulin. Of course, some patients do not comply with a healthy protocol, and in these cases, we rely on medication. The two most important supplements in managing Type II diabetes are chromium and vanadium (another trace mineral).

  A person doesn't suddenly develop Type II diabetes. The condition starts out as hypoglycemia (low blood sugar), followed by hyperglycemia (high sugar and high insulin levels); in time, the pancreas becomes fatigued and releases little or no insulin, along with high blood sugar levels. Once the pancreas has been damaged, you may need medication or insulin, or both. Ideally, the problem can be addressed early, in the hypoglycemic phase, before there are complications. Once full-blown Type II diabetes has developed, the condition can still be controlled, but it will take more effort.

R_x FOR HEALTH

FOR ALL DIABETICS

Lifestyle
- Maintain a healthy weight. Most diabetics weigh thirty to sixty pounds more than they should. For more information on weight loss, see Chapter 7, "Reshaping Your Body," page 115.

- Exercise regularly. Studies have shown that vigorous exercise can lower the risk of developing Type II diabetes by one-third. (Strive to work in the exercise benefit zone; see page 134 for more information.)

Diet

- Eliminate all sugar and processed carbohydrates from the diet.

- Eat a diet high in soluble fiber, which has been shown to help keep blood sugar under control and slow down the absorption of food. Beans (all types) are an excellent source of soluble fiber. Soluble fiber supplements are also available from health food stores.

- Consume 10 grams of pectin (or 5 grams of the plant fiber guar) with meals. These plant fibers help reduce insulin requirements. Apples and citrus fruits are an excellent source of pectin, but you need commercial supplements to get really effective amounts.

Nutritional Supplements

The following supplements should be taken as a maintenance dose on an ongoing basis. Take supplements five days, then take the weekends off.

- Take a complete vitamin/mineral supplement each day. (See Chapter 9, "Enough Is Not Always Enough," page 149 for more information on nutritional supplements.)

- Take 250 milligrams of vitamin C once a day to reduce oxidative damage.

- Take 300 milligrams of magnesium daily. Many diabetics have a deficiency in magnesium; supplements, even at low doses, tend to minimize complications related to the disease.

- Take 5 to 15 milligrams of zinc daily. This mineral helps with insulin production; it can be poorly absorbed by the digestive tract, so supplementation is important.

Herbs

The following herbs can be used alone or in combination for up to two weeks at a time during periods of emotional or physical stress.

- Garlic. This herb helps lower blood sugar levels. The active agents appear to be acyl propyl disulfide and allicin. Eat 3 to 6 cloves of garlic a day, or use commercially prepared products and follow package directions.

- Onion. Onions have been shown to have a significant blood sugar–lowering effect. Dose: 50 to 150 grams of commercially prepared extract per day; follow package directions.

- Ginseng. This herb helps to reduce blood sugar levels. Commercial products are available at health food stores.

- Sage. Studies show that sage lowers blood sugar levels when consumed on an empty stomach. For an infusion, use 1 to 2 teaspoons of dried leaves per cup of boiling water; steep for 10 minutes. Drink up to 3 cups a day.

- Fenugreek. Studies have shown that this herb can reduce urine sugar levels by 50 percent. For a decoction, gently boil 2 teaspoons of bruised seeds per cup of water; simmer 10 minutes, strain, and drink up to 3 cups a day.

FOR TYPE I DIABETICS

Diet
- Avoid dairy products for the first six months after you have been diagnosed with the disease. Have your doctor perform an evaluation to see if you have a dairy allergy.

Nutritional Supplements
- Take 1 gram of niacinamide twice a day for the first twelve months after the diabetes is diagnosed.

- Take 400 to 800 IU of vitamin E daily. This antioxidant helps reduce inflammation. Take it as a maintenance supplement on an ongoing basis; take it for five days, then take weekends off.

FOR TYPE II DIABETICS

The following supplements can be taken as a maintenance dose on an ongoing basis. Take supplements five days, then take weekends off.

Nutritional Supplements

- Take 200 micrograms of chromium twice a day. Studies have found that people with adult-onset diabetes can lower their insulin requirements by taking chromium supplements. Chromium, an essential micronutrient, makes insulin about ten times more efficient at processing sugar, so less insulin is needed to do the job. Unfortunately, levels of chromium in the body tend to decrease with age. Instead of taking a supplement of chromium picolonate or chromium chloride, you can take it in the form of 9 grams of brewer's yeast daily.

  NOTE: A doctor should monitor the impact of chromium supplementation on the body since large fluctuations in blood glucose levels should be avoided.

- Take 5 to 10 milligrams of vanadium three times a day.

- Take 5 milligrams of manganese twice a day.

- Take 10 milligrams of biotin twice a day.

FOR COMPLICATIONS WITH TYPE I
OR TYPE II DIABETES

- If you have vision complications, take the following supplements on an ongoing basis. Take supplements five days, then take weekends off:

  - Take 40 to 60 milligrams of bilberry twice a day.

  - Take 500 milligrams of quercitin twice a day.

- Take 250 milligrams of taurine twice a day.

- Take a B-complex-25 (25 milligrams of each B vitamin) twice a day.

- If you have kidney complications, take the following supplements on an ongoing basis. Take supplements five days, then take weekends off:

  - Avoid nonsteroidal anti-inflammatory drugs (such as aspirin, Motrin, and so on).

  - Be sure to drink an adequate amount of water (at a minimum, eight 8-ounce glasses a day).

  - Take 1 gram of fish oil twice a day.

  - Take 240 milligrams of GLA (gammalinolenic acid) twice a day (as evening primrose oil).

- If you have nerve problems, take the following supplements on an ongoing basis. Take supplements five days, then take weekends off:

  - Take 2 grams of fish oil three times a day.

  - Take 240 milligrams of GLA (gammalinolenic acid) three times a day.

  - Take 50 milligrams of vitamin B_6 twice a day.

  - Take 50 milligrams of pycnogenol twice a day.

- If you have cardiovascular complications, take the following supplements on an ongoing basis. Take supplements five days, then take weekends off:

  - Take 400 to 800 IU of vitamin E daily. This vitamin helps the body maintain normal glucose or blood sugar levels.

  - Take 500 milligrams of taurine twice a day.

  - Take 200 micrograms of selenium daily.

▼▼▼▼▼▼▼▼▼▼▼▼▼▼▼▼▼▼▼▼▼▼▼▼

ACUPUNCTURE AND PAIN CONTROL

If nerve damage occurs as a complication of diabetes, acupuncture can be helpful in pain control. A fifty-five-year-old African American woman developed severe nerve damage in the left side of her chest and abdomen as a complication of diabetes. The excruciating pain left her nauseated, and the abdominal pain made eating all but impossible. She visited multiple physicians, but no one was able to help her. She then came to us and we encouraged her to try acupuncture. After several sessions, she was able to enjoy food again; after a few months of treatment, her pain disappeared. For the past four years, she has remained pain-free, though she must still take other steps to control the diabetes.

▲▲▲▲▲▲▲▲▲▲▲▲▲▲▲▲▲▲▲▲▲▲▲▲

▼▼▼▼▼▼▼▼▼▼▼▼▼▼▼▼▼▼▼▼▼▼▼▼

OUR HISTORY OF HEALING

Bitter melon or balsam pear is a tropical vegetable grown in Africa that is used as a folk medicine remedy for diabetes. The blood sugar–lowering action of the fresh juice of the unripe fruit has in fact been clearly established in both experimental and clinical studies. Bitter melon contains several compounds with confirmed antidiabetic properties. Charantin, extracted by alcohol, contains anti-inflammatory compounds that are more potent than the drug tolbutamide, which is often used in the treatment of diabetes. Studies have found that people who drink 50 to 60 milliliters of bitter melon juice have positive results, though we have not tried it in our practice.

▲▲▲▲▲▲▲▲▲▲▲▲▲▲▲▲▲▲▲▲▲▲▲▲

▼▼▼▼▼▼▼▼▼▼▼▼▼▼▼▼▼▼▼▼▼▼▼▼▼▼▼

FOR MORE INFORMATION

American Diabetes Association
National Center
P.O. Box 25757
1660 Duke Street
Alexandria, VA 22314
(703) 549-1500
(800) ADA-DISC

Diabetes Research Institute Foundation
3440 Hollywood Blvd., Suite 100
Hollywood, FL 33021
(305) 964-4040

International Diabetes Center
3800 Park Nicollet Blvd.
Minneapolis, MN 55416
(612) 927-3393

Joslin Diabetes Center
One Joslin Place
Boston, MA 02215
(617) 732-2415

National Diabetes Information Clearinghouse
Box NDIC
9000 Rockville Pike
Bethesda, MD 20892
(301) 468-2162

▲▲▲▲▲▲▲▲▲▲▲▲▲▲▲▲▲▲▲▲▲▲▲▲▲▲▲

14

▼

An Ounce of Prevention

A Holistic Approach to Avoiding Cancer

We've been dealt a difficult hand: African Americans are more likely to get cancer, and more likely to die from it, than members of any other group in the United States. In the last forty years, the number of deaths from cancer has risen by 10 percent in the general population, but among African Americans the death toll has gone up by an astounding 50 percent.

Many of these deaths can be prevented. If African Americans receive timely medical care, many of those lives can be saved. While we do our best to keep our patients informed about cancer and its warning signs, the unfortunate reality is that most African Americans don't know the major warning signs of cancer. In fact, only 13 percent of all African Americans could identify a single cause of cancer, according to the National Medical Association, a medical society of black doctors. In addition, compared to people of other races, African Americans tend to have fewer screening tests done, receive less information about the link between lifestyle choices and cancer, and are exposed to more carcinogens at work and at home.

In addition, there is another factor at work, one that cannot be summed up in a survey or neatly measured in a clinical study. It is the problem of hopelessness and the link between despair in the soul and disease in the body. A growing body of literature—as well as our decades of experience as physicians treating people with cancer—supports the idea that psychological factors can play an important role in the development and treatment of cancer.

Most of our patients are astounded when we tell them that our bodies produce cancer cells all the time. They become nervous, then relax when we explain that in most cases, a healthy immune system and the body's natural killer cells destroy these deviant cells before they spread. It takes both the existence of cancer cells and the failure of the immune system for the cancer to take hold.

The mind can have a powerful influence over the immune system; there is even evidence to support the notion of a cancer-type personality. In fact, researchers have found that cancer is more common in people who do not have loving relationships and in those who tend to internalize their emotions. Sometimes these people seem nice—or overly nice—but just below the surface there is anger, even rage. Often when these people experience a major disappointment, perhaps a death, divorce, or a problem at work, they feel hopeless and depressed. This change in their emotional state can weaken the immune system and give the cancer a foothold. In the same way, the independent thinkers who refuse to accept cancer and who willingly fight for their health do in fact tend to do better battling the disease.

We have also seen patients who have been transformed by the process of being sick. In many of these cases, it seems as though the patients need to experience illness so that they can give themselves permission to play and enjoy life. Once these people become sick, they often begin to live in the moment; once they realize that their lives are finite, it becomes easier for them to play, to forgive, to dance, to enjoy.

The implications of this mind-body link should not be taken lightly; we believe it will be the key to cancer treatment in the future. Thoughts and behaviors that weaken the immune system can allow cancers to spread just as thoughts and behaviors that strengthen the immune system can help control the spread of some types of cancers. We are not saying that all cancers can be controlled by the mind alone—that can lead to a lot of blaming the patient—but rather that you can use the power of your mind to strengthen your immune system and improve your chances of managing the cancer.

This may sound far-fetched to people accustomed to dealing with

Western medicine, but we have seen the mind-body link established time and again in our practices. One woman had breast cancer, and new tumors would form each time she experienced a major life change—when her children left home or when she had difficulties with her spouse, for example. We have also had patients with cancers considered incurable who went through spiritual and physical cleansing and found their tumors shrinking in size. We do not understand the power of our minds, but we must respect the body's almost unlimited ability to heal itself.

A SHORT PRIMER ON CANCER

Every day your body produces more than 500 billion new cells. Most of the time the system works, but periodically an error occurs and a defective cell is created. This single cell can mark the beginning of cancer.

Cancerous tumors grow when a carcinogen (a cancer-causing agent) damages the genes that control cell growth. Most of the time, the body's immune system searches out and destroys these defective cells before they multiply, but if the immune system isn't doing its job, the cancer cells reproduce and form a tumor. In time, the tumor invades healthy tissue, stealing away nutrients from the body and damaging the body's organs.

While all cancers involve the uncontrolled growth of cells, *cancer* is actually a term that refers to more than a hundred different diseases. There are four main categories of cancer: **carcinomas** of the skin, mucous membranes, glands, and other organs; **leukemia** of the blood; **sarcomas** of the muscles, connective tissues, and bones; and **lymphomas** of the lymphatic system.

Not all tumors are cancerous: Benign (noncancerous) tumors do not spread to the surrounding tissue; malignant (cancerous) tumors do spread (or metastasize) through the blood vessels and lymph system to other areas of the body, where new tumors grow. Areas of the body where malignant tumors most commonly develop are the bone marrow, breasts, colon, liver, lungs, lymphatic system, ovaries, pancreas, prostate, skin, stomach, and uterus.

While many types of cancer can be treated—especially if detected at the earliest stages—the disease varies greatly in its aggressiveness.

Natural remedies can help to bolster the body's defense mechanisms and restore its natural healing processes, but there are no "cures" that promise to work all of the time.

The key to managing cancer is preventing it, and one of the keys to cancer prevention is a strong immune system. Unfortunately, in the decades that we have been practicing medicine, we have seen a steady decline in immune function among African Americans. We have seen a deterioration in the diets consumed by many African Americans, who eat more refined carbohydrates and trans-fats than ever before. We have seen an increase in the daily levels of stress faced by African Americans, who must contend with racial, financial, workplace, and social stresses. And we have seen an erosion in the spiritual support provided by African American communities, where churches and religious institutions once played a primary role in how we deal with our perception of injustice and prejudice.

All of these factors have taken a toll on our health. We have seen an alarming increase in the number of African American patients who develop chronic immune dysfunction disorders, such as chronic fatigue syndrome, skin problems, allergies, and cancer. Many factors tend to undermine and weaken the immune system, leaving us susceptible to illness and infection. Consider this partial list of immune-system suppressors (some we can control, others we can't):

> aging (your immune system starts slipping at age thirty)
> alcohol use
> allergies (first they stimulate immune activity, then they
>   suppress it)
> anti-inflammatory drugs
> antibiotics
> bacteria
> caffeine
> chemotherapy and radiation treatments
> depression and loneliness
> dietary problems, including a high-sugar, high-fat, low-protein diet
> excess dietary iron
> fungi
> industrial chemicals

insulin
lack of exercise
lack of sleep or rest
low self-esteem
parasites
pesticides
photochemical smog
recreational drug use
steroids
stress and emotional upset
surgery
travel
viruses
vitamin deficiencies, especially deficiencies in vitamins A, C, and E,
    the B vitamins, selenium, and zinc

These immune-system suppressors not only contribute to a weakened immune system, but they can also trigger hyperimmunity or autoimmunity disorders, in which the immune system malfunctions and attacks itself. (Examples of this include rheumatoid arthritis, erythematosis, and thyroiditis, among others.) Of course, maintaining a healthy immune system cannot prevent all disease and immune disorders, but it can go a long way toward avoiding many health problems.

THE BEST OFFENSE

The best approach to cancer is prevention. Some people inherit a predisposition toward cancer; others increase their risk of developing the disease through the lifestyle choices they make. Your cancer-fighting strategy for health is essentially a strategy for healthy living. To be healthy, you need a healthy immune system, supported by a positive attitude, healthy lifestyle, and appropriate care and maintenance of your body. We remind our patients of these common cancer prevention Do's and Don'ts:

- **DON'T smoke.** Cigarette smoking has been linked to lung cancer as well as cancers of the mouth, throat, and larynx. Pipe and cigar smoking contributes to mouth and throat cancer as well. If you smoke, one of the most obvious ways to reduce your cancer risk—as well as your risk of many other medical problems—is to kick the habit.

- **DO avoid exposure to known or suspected carcinogens at work and at home.** Whenever possible, avoid cleaning chemicals (especially those used in dry cleaning), coal tar, asbestos, gasoline, and petroleum products. If you suspect a chemical may compromise your health, behave as though it does. Check your home for radon gas (which has been linked to lung cancer) and avoid unnecessary X rays.

- **DO limit your fat intake.** A high-fat diet, especially a diet high in saturated animal fats, increases your risk of developing cancer of the breast, colon, prostate, uterus, or ovaries. Rancid oil and foods fried in oil produce damaging free radicals, which can contribute to cancer. Avoid meat and dairy products, fried foods, rancid oils, and hydrogenated and partially hydrogenated oils. (For more information on dietary fat, see Chapter 5, "Back into Balance," page 85.)

- **DO maintain a healthy weight.** Obesity (being more than 20 percent above your ideal body weight) is linked to colon, rectal, and prostate cancers in men, and breast, cervical, uterine, ovarian, and gallbladder cancer in women.

- **DO undergo early screening tests as part of your regular health care.** See the chart of screening tests in Chapter 1 on page 10.

- **DO avoid excessive exposure to sunlight.** The radiation from the sun has been linked to skin cancer, even among African Americans. When you spend time outdoors—especially during the peak hours of 10 A.M. to 2 P.M.—wear a wide-brimmed hat, sunglasses, tightly woven clothing, and a broad-spectrum sunscreen with a skin protection factor (SPF) of 15 or higher that blocks both UV-A and UV-B rays. Also wear SPF 15 lip balm; the lips are a common site for skin cancer.

- **DO get regular exercise.** You need to keep moving to stay resistant to infection and to keep the nutrients and immune components circulating through the body. The body's lymphatic system helps to remove foreign cells and proteins from the body by moving them to the blood, where they can be attacked, broken down, and eliminated. The lymphatic system is a circulatory system with no pump; it needs muscular activity to keep it moving. A sedentary lifestyle leads to a sluggish lymphatic system, and an increased likelihood of infections and immune-related illness. (You've probably felt the lymph nodes in your neck swell when you have a cold or flu; lymph nodes are storage stations for lymph cells along the lymphatic pathways. When the body encounters infection, the nodes closest to the infection site often swell and become tender. While hundreds of lymph nodes exist on the body, the best known are in the neck and groin, though the tonsils, adenoids, and appendix are lymphatic tissues as well.)

- **DO drink filtered or purified water.** In many cities, tap water contains heavy metals, pesticides, vinyl chloride, carbon tetrachloride, gasoline, and other known and suspected carcinogens. You need the water but not the contaminants.

- **DO practice safer sex by using barrier forms of contraception.** Researchers have proved a link between the human papilloma virus (which causes venereal warts) and cervical cancer in women.

- **DO work on developing psychological fitness.** Strive to build a network of social, emotional, and spiritual support. Studies have found that people with a strong support network tend to have a better prognosis than those who go it alone. If you are confronted with difficult life issues and decisions that you need to talk over with someone, reach out for help. Being able to express negative emotions and seek psychological support can help stabilize your physical as well as your mental health.

- **DO take time to rest or reflect.** Get enough sleep and take time to go inside yourself during the day. Breathe; meditate; let go of the tension of the day. (See Chapter 4, "Attitude Is Everything," page 59, for more information on relaxation.) Being well rested emotionally helps relieve stress and facilitate proper metabolism; it also helps stimulate the production of two important immune-system components, interleukin and interferon.

▼▼▼▼▼▼▼▼▼▼▼▼▼▼▼▼▼▼▼▼▼▼▼▼▼

OUR HERITAGE OF HEALING

In equatorial Africa, colon cancer is rare among the native people. Why? In the tropical African countries from Uganda to Ghana, high-fiber starchy roots are a dietary staple, much as the white potato is in the typical American diet. The dietary fiber helps cleanse the digestive system and keep it healthy, naturally.

▲▲▲▲▲▲▲▲▲▲▲▲▲▲▲▲▲▲▲▲▲▲▲▲▲

R$_x$ for Health

NOTE: To minimize the risk of developing cancer, the National Cancer Institute recommends that all Americans eat at least five to nine servings of fruits and vegetables daily, but only 9 percent of Americans heed this advice. According to experts at the NCI, as many as 50 percent of all cancers could be prevented by eating the right foods.

In addition to the Do's and Don't listed above, consider using the following recommendations:

Diet
- **Eat allium vegetables.** More than five hundred plants belong to the genus *Allium,* including garlic, onions, chives, and scallions. Use these vegetables liberally in your cooking. Garlic and onion are both rich in quercetin and selenium, two antioxidants that may play an important role in cancer prevention. Odorless garlic capsules are commercially available; follow package directions.

- **Eat a diet rich in high beta-carotene foods.** This powerful antioxidant helps destroy cancer-causing free radicals in the body. Low blood levels of beta-carotene have been linked to an increased risk of different types of cancer, especially breast, bladder, colon, and lung cancer. Foods high in beta-carotene include apricots, broccoli, cantaloupe, carrots, mangoes, peaches, pumpkin, spinach, and sweet potatoes.

- **Eat cruciferous vegetables every day.** Epidemiological studies have shown that people who eat a diet high in cruciferous vegetables (such as broccoli, Brussels spouts, cabbage, cauliflower, and kale) have lower rates of cancer than people who don't. Researchers have found that these vegetables contain indoles and sulforaphane, phytochemicals that help fight cancer. Eat at least two ½-cup servings of these vegetables every day; broccoli sprouts are an exceptionally good source of cancer-fighting nutrients.

- **Eat at least one ½-cup serving of fruits containing ellagic acid every day.** Animal studies have found that ellagic acid, a polyphenolic compound found in fruit, counteracts carcinogens, preventing healthy cells from becoming cancerous. Ellagic acid is also an antioxidant, which blocks the negative effects of free radicals. Strawberries, grapes, and cherries are good sources of ellagic acid.

- **Eat 30 to 35 grams of fiber a day.** A high-fiber diet helps to deter a number of different types of cancer, including breast and colon cancer. Eating a low-fiber diet slows the transit time for food to travel through the intestine, giving carcinogens a longer time to irritate the lining of the intestinal tract. The result: Low-fiber diets have been linked to high rates of colon cancer. Studies have shown that women who eat wheat bran regularly have low blood estrogen levels; high blood estrogen levels have been linked to cancer. The recommended 30 to 35 grams of fiber can be found in a diet including at least five servings of fruits and vegetables daily combined with roughly six servings of whole grains.

- **Eat soy-based foods daily.** Genistein, an ingredient in soy and soy-based products, appears to prevent the growth of cancerous tumors by inhibiting the formation of the blood vessels necessary to nourish them. For example, studies show that the rate of prostate cancer is the same in Japanese and American men, but the cancers grow much more slowly in Japanese men, who eat a diet rich in genistein. Good sources of genistein include whole soybeans, tofu, soy flour, soy milk, and rehydrated vegetable proteins (but not soy sauce).

- **Eat at least one serving of lutein-rich vegetables a day.** Lutein is found in fruits and vegetables in the carotenoid family; epidemiological studies have linked a high intake of fruits and vegetables rich in carotenoids with a lower risk of cancer. Carotenoids give fruits and vegetables their orange, red, and yellow colors; they are also found in green leafy vegetables, although the color is masked by the green from the chlorophyll. Foods rich in lutein include broccoli, carrots, celery, collard greens, green beans, kale, peas, spinach, turnip greens, and yams.

- **Eat at least one lycopene-rich food a day.** Lycopene is a phytochemical found in fruits and vegetables in the carotenoid family. Lycopene gives fruits and vegetables their reddish color; it is found in red peppers, ruby red grapefruit, and tomatoes. Studies have shown a link between low blood levels of lycopene and increased risk of bladder and pancreatic cancer. Commercial preparations are also available; follow package directions.

- **Eat at least one quercetin-rich food a day.** Quercetin is a bioflavonoid found in fruits and vegetables. Studies have shown that quercetin blocks cancer cell development; epidemiological studies have also shown that people who eat a diet rich in onions tend to develop fewer gastrointestinal cancers. Some of the best food sources of quercetin are broccoli, yellow and red onions, shallots, and zucchini.

- **Skip the sugar.** Sugar may be sweet to eat, but it is murder on the immune system. Studies have shown that eating 100 grams of simple sugars—glucose, fructose, honey, or fruit juice—can suppress the immune system for up to five hours, including the ability of the white blood cells to kill bacteria and viruses. If you check product labels, you may be surprised at the sugar content of many foods. For example, a single 12-ounce can of sugared cola contains about 40 milligrams of sugar, an 8-ounce glass of either orange juice or skim milk contains 25 milligrams of sugar, and ½ cup of spaghetti sauce includes about 13 grams of sugar.

Nutritional Supplements

The following supplements can be taken as a preventive dose on an ongoing basis. Take supplements five days, then take the weekends off.

- **Take 250 milligrams of calcium and 500 milligrams of magnesium daily.** Several studies have linked low intake of calcium with an increased risk of colon cancer. One study found that a daily intake of just 375 milligrams of calcium (approximately the amount in one 8-ounce glass of milk) was associated with a 50-percent reduction in the rate of colon cancer, and consuming 1200 milligrams of calcium was linked to a 75-percent decrease in colon cancer. Researchers speculate that the calcium binds with fatty acids, preventing them from irritating the colon walls. The low intake of calcium may also increase the rate of excretion of vitamin D, which also appears to play a role in helping to prevent colon cancer. The magnesium is necessary to balance the calcium and to avoid overstimulating the nervous system.

- **Take coenzyme Q-10 daily.** Every cell in the body contains coenzyme Q-10, a protein that works with other enzymes to provide the cells with energy. Coenzyme Q-10 inhibits the formation of free radicals, unstable oxygen molecules that can cause cellular damage and cancer. It is commercially available in capsule form; follow package directions.

- **Take one dose of flaxseed oil daily.** Studies have shown that people who consume diets rich in flax have lower levels of breast cancer. Flax contains an ingredient (lignans) that deactivates estrogens that cause certain tumors to grow; these lignans bind to estrogen receptor sites on cells in place of the more potent estrogens. Flaxseed oil is available in capsule and liquid form at natural food stores; follow package directions. Look for products with stabilized flax, since ordinary flax becomes rancid quickly. Keep flaxseed oil refrigerated to prevent it from spoiling.

- **Take 400 to 800 micrograms of folic acid daily.** Studies have found that people who eat low levels of folic acid tend to have high rates of precancerous tumors of the colon and rectum.

- **Take up to 500 milligrams of L-arginine daily.** This nonessential amino acid can stimulate the release of growth hormone produced by the pituitary gland in the brain. Animal studies have found that L-arginine helps inhibit the growth of tumors. Studies with human blood cells show that L-arginine increases the production of immune cells that interfere with tumor growth. In addition to nutritional supplements, try to include foods high in L-arginine. Good food sources of L-arginine include brown rice, popcorn (no butter), raisins, nuts, and sesame and sunflower seeds.

- **Take 1 gram of fish oil daily.** In the 1970s, scientists noticed that although Eskimos consumed large amounts of fat, they had an exceptionally low rate of heart disease and cancer. The fat in the Eskimo diet took the form of omega-3 fatty acids, which are found primarily in marine plant life phytoplanktons that are eaten by fatty fish. A number of animal studies have found that omega-3 fatty acids delay the onset of tumors and decrease the rate of growth, size, and number of tumors in animals in which cancer was induced. Good food sources include salmon, mackerel, albacore tuna, halibut, and sardines; eat two or three servings a week. While most researchers believe omega-3 fatty acids are most effective when consumed as foods, the fish oil is also available in capsule form. NOTE: Be cautious about taking omega-3 supplements if you are taking anticoagulants or taking aspirin daily, since excessive amounts of the oils can thin the blood. Discuss the matter with your doctor or health care provider.

- **Take 50 to 300 micrograms of selenium daily.** Broad-based epidemiological studies have shown that the mineral selenium may protect against certain cancers, particularly breast, colon, and lung cancer. Selenium inactivates peroxides in the cells, which can result in tissue damage. Dietary selenium is found in seafood, organ meats, and whole grains. NOTE: Most vitamin and mineral combination supplements do not contain selenium.

- **Take one teaspoon of tocotriene once a day.** Tocotrienols are the antioxidants and other nutrients found in rice bran. Ferulic acid (found in rice bran) has been found to block the formation of cancer-causing nitrosamines in the body. Because the cancer-fighting nutrients in rice bran are destroyed by cooking, we recommend that our patients take commercially prepared tocotriene. This supplement can be hard to find, but a stabilized form of tocotriene is available from The African American Product Company/Nia (a word meaning "purpose" in Swahili), 888-313-3103.

- **Take up to 1500 milligrams of vitamin C daily in divided doses.** This powerful antioxidant has been shown to protect against breast cancer in postmenopausal women; studies have also shown that taking as much as 3 grams of vitamin C a day reduces the number of rectal polyps, which have been associated with colon cancer. In addition, it appears to protect against stomach cancer by blocking the formation of nitrosamines, which are potential carcinogens. Vitamin C helps white blood cells function, and it increases the production of interferon, a substance suspected of helping to ward off cancer.

- **Take 400 to 800 IU of vitamin E a day.** A deficiency in vitamin E has been linked to breast cancer. It may also help to prevent stomach cancer and other cancers of the gastrointestinal tract by inhibiting the conversion of nitrates in foods to nitrosamines, which are potential carcinogens. NOTE: Be cautious about taking supplemental vitamin E if you are taking a blood thinner or have a bleeding problem.

▼▼▼▼▼▼▼▼▼▼▼▼▼▼▼▼▼▼▼▼▼▼▼▼▼▼▼

Key Cancer-Fighting Herbs

The following herbs can be used to bolster the immune system in patients with cancer. Consider using one or more of the herbs on an ongoing basis if you have been diagnosed with cancer. As a preventive measure, use the herbs for two weeks at a time four times a year at the change of seasons.

- *Red clover (Trifolium pratense).* For more than a hundred years, herbalists have used red clover to treat cancer. The herb contains several tumor-fighting compounds, as well as antioxidants. However, it should not be used on estrogen-dependent cancers, such as breast cancer. For an infusion, use 1 to 3 teaspoons of dried flowertops per cup of boiling water. Steep 10 to 15 minutes, strain, and drink up to 3 cups a day. Commercially prepared products are also available; follow package directions.

- *Ginkgo (Ginkgo biloba).* Ginkgo is rich in antioxidants that protect the body against free radicals, which damage healthy cells and can cause cancer. Ginkgo is not widely available as a bulk herb, but commercial preparations are available; follow package directions.

- *Ginseng (Panax quinquefolius).* Studies have shown that certain compounds in ginseng (saponins) stopped the growth of some cancer cells in animal studies. The herb also stimulates the immune system. Ginseng must be prepared properly for it to be mature and useful; look for commercial herbs or preparations made from whole, unprocessed, six-year-old roots. (It should say so on the label.) Follow package directions.

▲▲▲▲▲▲▲▲▲▲▲▲▲▲▲▲▲▲▲▲▲▲▲▲▲

▼▼▼▼▼▼▼▼▼▼▼▼▼▼▼▼▼▼▼▼▼▼▼

WATCH OUT!

While many cancers grow undetected in the body for months, years, or decades before making themselves known, watch out for these common symptoms or warning signs of different types of cancer:

a lump under the skin

persistent cough or chronic hoarseness

coughing up bloody sputum

difficulty swallowing

chronic indigestion

a thickening or lump in the breast (usually in the outer or upper part of the breast); there may be dimpling or creasing of the skin near the lump

discharge from the nipple

bleeding or discharge, bleeding between menstrual periods

painful or heavy menstrual periods

obvious changes in bowel or bladder habits

blood in the stool or urine

a persistent low-grade fever

headaches accompanied by visual disturbances

fatigue

excessive bruising

repeated nosebleeds

loss of appetite and weight loss

change in size or shape of the testes

persistent abdominal pain

continuous unexplained pain in the back or pelvis

a sore or ulceration that does not heal

a change in a wart or mole; pay special attention to the ABCD rule:

- Asymmetry: Moles are symmetrical, cancers are not.
- Borders: Moles have smooth borders, cancers have irregular or poorly defined borders.
- Color: Variation in either shade or color from one area of the mole to another is a warning sign, as is the presence of red, white, or blue.
- Diameter: Moles larger than six millimeters (roughly the size of a pencil eraser) should be checked by a dermatologist.

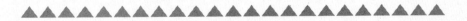

15

▼

Women's Bodies, Women's Health

Exploring What It Means to Be Black, Female, and Healthy

Back in 1983, more than two thousand women gathered at Spelman College in Atlanta to attend the first National Conference on Black Women's Health Issues. While this was not the first conference ever held on African American health, it may have been the first conference designed to encourage African American women to join together to discuss their unique health care needs. We strongly support organizations dedicated to women's health, and in our practices we strive to respect and appreciate the health care needs of women.

From the moment of conception to the moment of death, a woman's reproductive hormones create subtle—and sometimes not so subtle—changes in her body. Certain landmark events such as the onset of menstruation, pregnancy, and menopause present clear evidence of a woman's changing body. Other health care concerns such as breast lumps, osteoporosis, and vaginal dryness are triggered by hormone changes, though the hormonal links are less obvious.

In this chapter, we will touch on several of the common problems our female patients discuss with us. The first section covers concerns during the reproductive years; the second part looks at problems associated with menopause. In each section, we will describe some of the remedies that we have found to work with our patients. Due to the complexities of the human body and reproductive system, not every remedy will work with every woman every time. Please consult a health care professional if your symptoms persist after trying these remedies for several weeks.

CHALLENGES OF THE CHILDBEARING YEARS

To every season, there are unique health care needs. During a woman's fertile years, she experiences monthly fluctuations in her hormones that change with the phases of the menstrual cycle. These changes can result in premenstrual syndrome, painful cramping during menstruation, and breast lumps. Bladder infections tend to be fairly common during this phase of life as well.

PMS

Premenstrual syndrome (PMS) is a very real problem that challenges many of our African American patients. More than 150 different symptoms have been associated with PMS, but the most common include breast tenderness, fatigue, bloating and weight gain, food cravings, anger, depression, and irritability. PMS occurs between ovulation and the start of the menstrual cycle, or about two weeks before monthly bleeding begins. Researchers have found that African American women tend to experience more of the emotional symptoms of PMS, while white women experience more of the physical symptoms. Many women suffer in silence, ashamed and embarrassed to talk about their feelings.

When women come to us with PMS, we try to help them reframe and redefine this premenstrual period as a sacred time of transition for the body to complete its monthly cycle. Our African ancestors recognized the importance of transition and even created rituals to help a person work from one stage of life to the next. While modern American culture tends not to ritualize change and transition, you can claim this experience for yourself and use it to help work through the monthly transitions of your menstrual cycle.

R℞ for Health

Nutritional Supplements

Use the following supplements in the two weeks before your menstrual period begins.

- **Take a 50-milligram B vitamin daily.** Vitamin B_6 helps clear water through the kidneys, helping to regulate hormone levels and remove toxins from the body. The complete B vitamin is necessary to keep all the B vitamins in balance.

- **Take 1500 milligrams of magnesium daily.** Some studies have shown that magnesium deficiency on a cellular basis correlates with PMS. To overcome this deficiency, take supplemental magnesium at amounts equal to or greater than the amount of calcium. During the premenstrual phase of your cycle (in the week before you begin to menstruate), take 1500 milligrams of magnesium and 750 milligrams of calcium. The higher levels of magnesium help to tranquilize the nerves and relax the muscles.

Herbal Remedies

- **Take 2 capsules of the herb angelica twice a day.** This herb is considered a female tonic. It can also be taken as tea. To prepare a tea, steep 1 teaspoon of dried herb in 1 cup of boiling water for 5 minutes. Strain and drink up to 3 cups a day.

▼▼▼▼▼▼▼▼▼▼▼▼▼▼▼▼▼▼▼▼▼▼▼▼▼

ARE YOUR DENTAL FILLINGS CAUSING THE PROBLEM?

The buildup of heavy metals in the body can cause emotional symptoms, such as those associated with PMS. Some European studies suggest that the mercury in dental amalgams (tooth filling materials) may leak out and accumulate in the body. Of course, not everyone should have all the mercury in their teeth removed, but if you have PMS or some other chronic medical issue, consult a dentist with expertise in this issue.

▲▲▲▲▲▲▲▲▲▲▲▲▲▲▲▲▲▲▲▲▲▲▲▲▲▲▲▲▲▲

MENSTRUAL CRAMPING

During or just before menstruation, many women experience muscle tension, cramping, and discomfort. In some cases, the pain is accompanied by nausea, vomiting, diarrhea, headache, dizziness, or blurred vision. The pain may involve the lower back, legs, or abdomen.

This condition is caused by overactive prostaglandins, the hormones that cause the uterus to contract during menstruation. Other contributing factors include lack of exercise and anxiety. The condition usually improves with age and after pregnancy, though in some cases the problem gets worse.

In some cases, painful periods can be caused by a physical problem, such as endometriosis, a sexually transmitted disease, pelvic inflammatory disease, or polyps. If you experience painful cramping, discuss the matter with your doctor to rule out any of these more serious primary problems. Regular exercise and avoiding obesity can solve the problem for many women. If the cramping is a normal part of how your body deals with menstruation, the following remedies may help.

℞ for Health

Use the following supplements and herbs on the days you experience cramping and discomfort.

Nutritional supplements
- **Take 1000 milligrams of evening primrose oil daily.** In the body, the evening primrose oil helps minimize inflammation.

Diet
- **Avoid eating foods high in saturated fats, animal foods, shellfish, and cheese, as well as foods and beverages containing**

caffeine. These foods can help make cramping worse. Instead, eat plenty of foods high in omega-3 fatty acids, such as salmon, trout, and flaxseed.

Herbal Remedies

- **Drink 3 cups of green tea daily.** Green tea contains ingredients that inhibit the cyclooxygenase enzyme, which contributes to the formation of the prostaglandins that cause cramping.

FIBROCYSTIC BREAST DISEASE

Many African American women have fibrocystic breast disease, or lumpy breasts. In most women, the lumps feel tender and vary in size at different stages of the menstrual cycle. The lumps are rubbery feeling, have smooth edges, and move freely underneath the skin. (As a general rule, cancerous lumps do not move, do not feel tender and smooth, and do not change in size with the menstrual cycle.) If you have any questions about a breast lump, immediately contact your health care provider to eliminate the possibility of breast cancer.

Breast lumps can be triggered by imbalances in the liver energy system caused by stress and emotional tension. The liver is essential in the conversion of hormones in the body; illness arises when the liver fails to keep the hormones in balance. In addition, foods that cause inflammation can contribute to fibrocystic breast disease; sweets are a common culprit and should be avoided.

℞ for Health

Make the following dietary changes and take the following supplements on an ongoing basis to reduce symptoms of fibrocystic breast disease.

Diet

- **Minimize your intake of saturated fat.** Nonorganic cattle and poultry are routinely fed hormones to improve their growth and milk production. These hormones often remain in the animal's flesh and tend to accumulate in the fats (including milk fats) that are passed on in the food we eat. Switching to a vegetarian or organic diet can sometimes cause breast lumps to disappear by themselves.

- **Eliminate caffeine from your diet.** Coffee, tea, chocolate, and other foods high in caffeine have been linked to lumpy breasts. Simply eliminating caffeine is enough to eliminate breast lumps for many women.

Nutritional Supplements

The following supplements can be taken every day for two to three months. After that time, take them for five days, then take weekends off.

- **Take 400 IU of vitamin E.** This powerful antioxidant helps reduce inflammation and prevent breast lumps.

- **Take a 50-milligram B-complex supplement daily.** This supplement helps to ensure that the body has enough folic acid and B vitamins to maintain balanced hormones.

- **Take 1000 milligrams of evening primrose oil three times a day.** This essential fatty acid helps to balance the hormones and eliminate breast lumps.

BLADDER INFECTIONS

Bladder infections or urinary tract infections occur almost thirty times more often in women than men. Many of these infections are caused by imbalances in the intestinal flora, especially after taking antibiotics or other drugs that disrupt the body's natural bacterial balance.

Other contributing factors can be birth control pills, a poorly fitting diaphragm, use of alcohol or caffeine, allergy to contraceptive spermicides, or frequent sexual activity. Women and girls should always wipe from front to back after bowel movements to avoid fecal contamination of the urethra, a source of bladder infections. The problem can be made worse by not drinking enough water or other fluids and by wearing tight pants or nylon underwear (which restrict air flow to the vagina and rub on the urethra).

Symptoms of bladder or urinary tract infection include a frequent urge to urinate, painful or burning urination, and pain or cramping in the pelvic area. The urine itself may appear cloudy or contain blood fragments. An untreated bladder infection can spread to the kidney, a more serious infection. Try the following remedies for two or three days; if symptoms persist, contact your doctor or health care provider.

℞ for Health

Nutritional Supplements

- **Take 1000 milligrams of vitamin C per hour with lots of water at the first sign of infection.** As soon as you experience the slightest suspicion that you may have a bladder infection, begin taking 1000 milligrams of vitamin C every hour for four or five hours. This may be enough to prevent the infection from taking hold; if not, it should cut short the course of the condition.

- **Take a *Lactobacillus acidophilus* supplement daily.** This bacterium helps fight infection and encourages the growth of beneficial bacteria in the digestive and urinary tracts. Commercial products are available; follow package directions.

Diet

- **Drink 3 cups of cranberry juice daily.** Cranberries really do help prevent and treat urinary tract infection. The berries contain a bacteria-fighting chemical known as hippuric acid. Drink 3 glasses of unsweetened cranberry juice a day for as long as necessary. You can also find concentrated cranberry pills at health food stores.

- **Drink 8 to 10 glasses of water a day.** The fluids help to flush the system and dilute the bacteria. When urine is left in the bladder, the bacteria have a chance to multiply.

Herbal Remedies

- **Take 3 doses of odorless garlic daily.** Garlic is a natural antibiotic. Odorless garlic capsules are commercially available.

- **Take 250 milligrams of goldenseal three times a day.** This herb helps to kill microbes, including the bacteria causing problems with a bladder infection.

THE CHALLENGES OF MENOPAUSE

At the most basic level, menopause is nothing more than the cessation of ovulation and menstrual cycles. It usually occurs in women between the ages of forty-five and fifty-five, with the average age being fifty-one. Most women experience irregular periods for five to seven years before their cycle stops entirely (this erratic time is known as perimenopause). A woman is considered to have passed through menopause after going one full year without menstrual periods.

During menopause, a number of changes take place in a woman's body in response to the changes in hormone levels. After the body stops producing estrogen, bones refuse to take in calcium (contributing to osteoporosis); a woman may experience night sweats, hot flashes, heart palpitations, insomnia, and emotional sensitivity due to fluctuations in hormone levels. Some women glide through menopause without symptoms or complaints; others experience a difficult transition. The discomforts of menopause tend to be especially severe if menstruation stops abruptly, either naturally or following surgical removal of the ovaries.

Hot flashes, a common menopausal complaint, occur when estrogen levels drop, causing a sudden adjustment in the body's thermostat and an abrupt "flash" of heat. The pituitary gland in the brain controls both the body's estrogen level and body temperature, hence the link between hormones and heat.

Typically the heat of a hot flash begins in the chest and spreads to the neck, face, and arms. It can be accompanied by sweating and heart palpitations, and it may be followed by chills. Three out of every four menopausal women experience hot flashes, which can occur as often as once an hour and can last for three or four minutes at a stretch.

To treat the complaints associated with menopause, many doctors prescribe synthetic hormones; we have found that most women can control the unpleasant side effects of menopause using natural medicine. Consider the fifty-one-year-old woman who came to the office to find out what her alternatives were to the synthetic hormones her doctor prescribed to control her menopausal symptoms. She had been relatively healthy throughout her life, but she experienced unpleasant hot flashes, night sweats, and irritability when she entered menopause. At times, the hot flashes were so severe that her husband had to leave the bed at night. She spoke to her gynecologist about her symptoms, and he prescribed the synthetic estrogen Premarin. The hot flashes stopped, but the woman started having uterine cramping and breakthrough bleeding. She gave up and stopped taking hormones.

When we saw her in the office, we reviewed her health history and carefully examined her diet. We recommended she increase her dietary protein, but we encouraged her to do this by increasing protein from nonanimal sources such as tofu and nuts rather than by eating more meat. We encouraged her to take two capsules of fish oil, 50 milligrams of zinc, and to eat three or four servings of beets each week. (Beets have a natural ability to flush the liver and enhance bile flow, which can help the body stabilize its hormone levels.) In four to six weeks, the woman's hot flashes resolved without the use of synthetic hormones. As this situation illustrates, many women's health problems can be traced back to hormone imbalances, many of which can be resolved without resorting to synthetic supplemental hormones.

However, some women need supplemental hormones, either because they are suffering from symptoms associated with hormone imbalances (hot flashes, vaginal dryness, moodiness, and so forth) or because they need the protection against osteoporosis and cardiovascular disease that estrogen provides. When women need supplemental hormones, we favor the use of natural progesterone (as a cream derived from wild yam); a woman's body can safely convert this to needed estrogen. We believe that most menopausal and postmenopausal women do not need estrogen; natural progesterone will safely and adequately do the trick. (Follow package directions for usage and dosage information.)

In menopause, estrogen drops to about one-third of premenopausal baseline levels, but progesterone typically drops to $\frac{1}{120}$ of the premenopausal level. We believe that the real hormonal problem women experience during menopause involves progesterone, not estrogen.

▼▼▼▼▼▼▼▼▼▼▼▼▼▼▼▼▼▼▼▼▼▼▼▼▼▼▼▼

BALANCED DIET, BALANCED HORMONES

A number of foods we eat contain phytoestrogens or plant estrogen, which can offer a natural dietary alternative to hormone therapy. Common foods, such as yams, soybeans, tofu, flaxseed, mangoes, millet, kale, and peanuts, contain estrogen-promoting compounds. In fact, phytoestrogens have been found in at least three hundred different plants.

▲▲▲▲▲▲▲▲▲▲▲▲▲▲▲▲▲▲▲▲▲▲▲▲▲▲▲▲

▼▼▼▼▼▼▼▼▼▼▼▼▼▼▼▼▼▼▼▼▼▼▼▼▼▼▼▼

THE GREAT HORMONE DEBATE

After menopause, should you take supplemental estrogen or not? There are trade-offs: Estrogen replacement therapy increases your risks of developing certain health problems, while lowering your risk of developing others.

When discussing hormone replacement with our female patients, we take the woman's specific risks and family medical history into account, of course. As you wrestle with the estrogen question, keep these pros and cons in mind:

The Pros

- **Estrogen protects against heart disease.** Heart disease and stroke kill more than half of all women over age fifty, more than all forms of cancer combined. Hormone replacement therapy lowers the risk of heart disease by about 50 percent by reducing levels of low-density lipoprotein cholesterol (the "bad" cholesterol) and increasing levels of high-density lipoprotein cholesterol (the "good" cholesterol). Simply being post-menopausal puts a woman at a higher risk for heart disease. If she has one additional risk factor—if she smokes, has high blood pressure, HDL cholesterol below thirty-five, diabetes, or family history of heart disease—she is at high risk for cardiovascular disease and should consider hormone therapy.

- **Estrogen helps prevent osteoporosis.** Hormone therapy lowers the risk of developing osteoporosis by slowing the rate of bone loss after menopause. Studies show that estrogen therapy can reduce the risk of osteoporosis fractures by up to 60 percent.

- **Hormone therapy may reduce the risk of developing Alzheimer's disease.** A recent study found that the longer a woman took estrogen, the lower her odds of getting Alzheimer's disease. For women who took hormones for ten years, the risk dropped by 30 to 40 percent.

- **Hormone therapy can ease common menopausal complaints.** Supplemental hormones can relieve hot flashes, vaginal dryness, mood swings, and other menopausal complaints associated with the fall in estrogen levels.

The Cons

- **Hormone replacement therapy may increase a woman's risk of developing breast cancer.** There is conflicting evidence about the link between hormones and breast cancer. While some studies show an increased cancer risk, others indicate that low doses of estrogen taken for less than five years do not increase breast cancer rates at all. To make matters more confusing, recent research by the American Cancer Society has shown that women who take synthetic hormones may be less likely to die from breast cancer, even if they are more likely to develop the disease. The study found that women who reported using estrogen for up to ten years had a 16-percent lower risk of dying from breast cancer, and those who began using estrogen before they were forty were 34 percent less likely to die from the disease.

Researchers speculate that the hormones may encourage the growth of slow-growing tumors and suppress the more aggressive and more deadly ones. Still, women at high risk of developing breast cancer may want to avoid additional estrogen, and all women taking estrogen should make a point to have an annual mammogram.

- **Estrogen may raise a woman's risk of developing endometrial cancer.** Studies suggest that hormone therapy increases the risk of developing endometrial cancer (cancer of the lining of the uterus). Combining estrogen and progestin (a synthetic form for the hormone progesterone) offsets the risk, but the addition of the progesterone reduces the cholesterol-reducing benefit of the estrogen.

- **Estrogen may make fibroids worse.** Estrogen can increase the size of fibroids (benign tumors in the uterus), causing bleeding and pain. Without supplemental estrogen, most fibroids shrink after menopause.

- **Hormones can cause gallstones.** Studies suggest that hormone replacement therapy more than doubles a woman's chances of developing gallstones.

- **Hormones can cause unpleasant side effects.** Hormone therapy can cause a number of unwelcome side effects, including hormone-related weight gain, fluid retention, nausea, headaches, breast tenderness, and regular monthly bleeding.

▲▲▲▲▲▲▲▲▲▲▲▲▲▲▲▲▲▲▲▲▲▲▲▲▲

Managing Menopausal Symptoms

Menopause is different for every woman. If your body can handle the hormonal ups and downs without distress, count your blessings. However, if you suffer from unpleasant side effects associated with menopause, consider experimenting with the following treatments.

R̽ for Health

Nutritional Supplements

Use these supplements as long as menopausal problems persist. Take the supplements and herbs for two weeks, then take one week off.

- **Take 500 milligrams of L-arginine and 500 milligrams of lysine twice a day.** These amino acids (taken on an empty stomach) help to detoxify the liver, which can help ease the symptoms associated with menopause.

- **Take 400 IU of vitamin E.** This antioxidant helps with all menopausal symptoms, including emotional upset. If you are taking supplemental estrogen, you need to take 800 IU daily.

- **Take 2 to 3 capsules of evening primrose oil daily.** Hot flashes respond well to evening primrose oil, which acts as a sedative and diuretic.

Diet

- **Avoid alcohol and caffeine.** Hot flashes can be exacerbated by alcohol (which opens the blood vessels) and caffeine (which is a stimulant). To minimize the chances of experiencing hot flashes, avoid both alcohol and caffeine.

- **Eat soy-rich foods.** Soybeans and other foods containing soy protein contain phytoestrogens, or molecules very similar to estrogen and progesterone. A menopausal woman who eats lots of soy protein can retain the benefits she had previously received from her body's natural estrogen. Try to consume 25 grams of soy daily; a soy burger contains about 18 grams, a glass of soy milk, about 8 grams. Powdered soy supplements, which can be mixed with milk or water, are also available at health food stores.

Herbal Remedies

- **Use black cohosh to control symptoms.** This herb has long been used to manage menopausal complaints due to its estrogenic effects, meaning it acts like the female hormone estrogen. Use a commercial product, following package directions. Or, for a decoction, boil ½ teaspoon of powdered root per cup of water for 30 minutes. Strain and drink 2 tablespoons every few hours, up to 1 cup a day.

- **Drink 2 cups of fenugreek tea a day.** Fenugreek seeds contain diosgenin, a chemical similar to the female hormone estrogen. Fenugreek tea is available at health food stores. To prepare a decoction, boil 2 teaspoons of seeds in 1 cup of water. Simmer for 10 minutes, strain, and drink up to 3 cups a day.

- **Use a commercial wild yam preparation.** This herb contains plant hormones very similar to the female hormone progesterone. In fact, until 1970, this plant was used in the manufacture of birth control pills. This herb is commercially available from health food stores. For more information on using natural progesterone, pick up a copy of the book *What Your Doctor May Not Tell You About Menopause,* by John R. Lee, M.D., and Virginia Hopkins (New York: Warner Books, 1996).

OSTEOPOROSIS

While osteoporosis can afflict anyone, it is actually much *less* common among African Americans than people of other races. After menopause, estrogen production declines, causing osteoporosis (a medical term that literally means "porous bones") in susceptible people. The thin, brittle bones associated with osteoporosis can lead to broken hips, vertebrae, and other bones.

In most cases, the problem arises when people consume too little calcium. The body needs this essential mineral for muscle contractions and other functions, so it "steals" from the bones, leaving them fragile and thin. Typically, women experience their peak bone mass in the spine at around age thirty and in the long bones at around age thirty-five. After that, bone mass drops by about 1 percent a year until menopause; after menopause, bone loss speeds up to about 2 to 4 percent a year for the next ten years or so.

African American women tend have thicker bones than people of other races, but other factors also play a role; smokers, alcoholics, diabetics, women who reach menopause before age forty, women who have never been pregnant, and those who consume a lot of caffeine are at increased risk of developing osteoporosis.

R̙ for Health

Nutritional Supplements

- **Take 1500 milligrams of calcium daily.** The primary cause of osteoporosis is calcium deficiency. Studies have shown that taking calcium supplements (with vitamin D) for only a year and a half dramatically decreases the number of bone fractures in women over age eighty. Women taking the supplements had 43 percent fewer hip fractures and 32 percent fewer fractures of the wrist, arm, and pelvis. You can also increase the calcium content on many foods you eat by adding powdered nonfat dry milk to recipes; every teaspoon of powdered milk adds about 50 milligrams of calcium. Calcium supplementation should be continued on an ongoing basis.

Lifestyle

- **Exercise for at least thirty minutes three times a week.** Regular weight-bearing exercise helps strengthen the bones. Aim for at least thirty minutes of exercise three or four times a week. Weight-bearing exercises include walking, jogging, cross-country skiing, bowling, dancing, weight lifting, tennis, and other activities that require you to support your body weight. (For more information on exercise, see Chapter 8, "Working It Out," page 127.)

Herbal Remedies

- **Drink 1 cup of horsetail tea daily.** This herb is good for bone repair. To make horsetail tea, simmer 2 teaspoons of the dried herb for 10 minutes in a cup of water. Steep for another 5 minutes, strain, and drink. Commercially prepared products are also available; follow package directions.

16
▼

Common Complaints

Living with Chronic Conditions

Chronic or recurring illnesses can be challenging to live with on a day-to-day basis. Some people find it almost impossible to escape the pain: Every morning, those with arthritis wake to stiff and achy joints; every night, those with insomnia anxiously lie in bed, waiting for sleep to come. Even when they are in periods of good health, patients with chronic health problems that come and go—such as asthma, migraine headaches, skin problems, and constipation—often feel anxious about the prospect of another episode of illness.

Managing an illness on an ongoing basis can be exasperating, and from time to time most of our patients with chronic ailments fall into a period of self-pity and complain, "It just isn't fair." They ask, "Why me? What did I do to deserve this ongoing pain?"

In these situations, we encourage those patients to reframe their illness, to view their chronic condition as a teacher, not as a punishment. As individuals, we have the ability to perceive our physical state in negative or positive terms. We challenge these patients to see their illness in a new way: Is there a lesson you can learn from this experience? Does the pain help you appreciate the many blessings you do have? Have you grown stronger by facing problems? Once they understand the power of reframing the illness, many of our patients view their chronic illness in a new light.

Of course, we also offer concrete advice on things that can be done to alleviate the symptoms and discomforts associated with a chronic condition. In this chapter, we will briefly describe a number of common chronic health problems that affect African Americans. Volumes could be written on natural remedies used for the treatment of these conditions, but we will focus on remedies that we have found helpful to a vast majority of our patients. If the natural remedies listed here do not help with your problem, please contact your health care provider for a more complete program of treatment.

ARTHRITIS: OSTEOARTHRITIS

Osteoarthritis is a degenerative joint disease that involves deterioration of the cartilage at the ends of the bones. It results in inflammation, pain, and stiffness, with weakening of the muscles, ligaments, and tendons. The onset can be sudden or gradual, and is most frequent after age forty, unless there has been earlier injury, excessive joint stress, or deformity from birth. Three times as many women as men suffer from osteoarthritis. The joints of the fingers, hips, knees, and spine are affected most often.

To create a smooth hinge between the bones, cartilage covers the ends of the bones and a membrane inside the joint secretes a lubricating gel known as synovial fluid; a gel-filled shell (the synovial joint) encloses the system. In a person with osteoarthritis, there may be too little synovial fluid in the joint, causing stiffness, or too much, causing swelling around the joint. If the cartilage at the ends of the bones is worn or chipped, the bone may scrape against bone, causing additional pain.

R̥ for Health

Nutritional Supplements
Take these supplements daily for six weeks. Then take them five days, with weekends off, as a maintenance dose.

- **Take 1500 milligrams of glucosamine and chondroitin sulfate.** As people age, their bodies produce less glucosamine and chondroitin sulfate, substances found inside the joints that help in the formation of cartilage. Without enough glucosamine and chondroitin, cartilage loses water and becomes a less effective cushion. Taking supplements helps reverse the effects of osteoarthritis. Glucosamine-chondroitin combination supplements are available at health food stores and from some physicians. Be sure to pick up a product containing glucosamine sulfate rather than glucosamine hydrochloride, since the research on effectiveness has been performed on the sulfate form.

- **Take 6 to 9 milligrams of boron.** Boron is necessary for the formation and maintenance of cartilage, but it is not included in many multiple vitamin/mineral supplements because the federal government has not established an RDA for the mineral. If you have osteoarthritis and your daily supplement does not include boron, take it as a separate supplement.

- **Take 1500 milligrams of vitamin C and 800 IU of vitamin E daily.** Both of these vitamins are powerful antioxidants, which help prevent damage to cartilage in the joints. Vitamin C also helps with the manufacture of collagen, a protein in cartilage; without enough vitamin C, the body stops producing collagen, and the joints become compromised.

Herbal Remedies

Use these herbs on an ongoing basis, taking them for five days, with weekends off.

- **Use the herb angelica to reduce pain and swelling.** Angelica's anti-inflammatory effects have made it a favorite arthritis treatment in Asian cultures for centuries. For a decoction, use 1 teaspoon of powdered root per cup of water. Bring to a boil, simmer 10 to 15 minutes, then remove from heat and let stand for 15 minutes. Drink up to 2 cups a day. Commercially prepared products are also available; follow package directions.

- **Take 2 grams of yucca leaves twice a day.** A chemical in the yucca plant (saponin) has been shown to help control osteoarthritis.

- **Take 2 grams of devil's claw twice a day.** This herb has both anti-inflammatory and analgestic effects; it contains a chemical, harpagoside, that reduces joint inflammation.

Diet
- **Avoid foods in the nightshade family.** Eliminating tomatoes, potatoes, eggplants, peppers—the so-called nightshade vegetables—can promote cartilage repair. Nightshade vegetables contain high levels of alkaloids, which may trigger joint problems in some people. The theory is that alkaloids remove calcium from the bones and deposit it in the joints, causing calcification, inflammation, and pain. An estimated 70 percent of arthritis sufferers who avoid nightshade-family vegetables report some relief from joint pain.

▼▼▼▼▼▼▼▼▼▼▼▼▼▼▼▼▼▼▼▼▼▼▼▼▼

PREVENTIVE CARE

To prevent the loss of cartilage in your joints, lose those extra pounds you've been carrying around. The more overweight you are, the more likely you are to develop osteoarthritis. (For more information on weight loss, see Chapter 7, "Reshaping Your Body," page 115.)

▲▲▲▲▲▲▲▲▲▲▲▲▲▲▲▲▲▲▲▲▲▲▲▲▲

▼▼▼▼▼▼▼▼▼▼▼▼▼▼▼▼▼▼▼▼▼▼▼▼▼

TREATING OSTEOARTHRITIS WITH HOMEOPATHY

Use one homeopathic treatment at a time, based on your specific symptoms. For information on homeopathy, see page 23. Discontinue use if the symptoms disappear.

- **Arnica** *(Arnica montana)* 30c. Use when joint pain is made worse by an injury, such as overuse. One dose four times a day, for up to four doses.

- **Bryonia** *(Bryonia alba* or *B. dioica)* 30c. Use for severe pain that feels worse with the slightest motion. The pain improves with cold and feels worse with heat treatment. One dose four times a day, for up to four doses.

- **Calcarea phos.** *(Calcarea phosphorica)* 6c. Use when affected joints feel numb and cold; symptoms become worse during weather changes. One dose four times a day, for up to two weeks.

- **Ledum** *(Ledum palustre)* 6c. Use when pain involves small joints, such as toes and fingers; the joints may crack and the pain may be relieved by cold treatment. One dose four times a day, for up to two weeks.

- **Rhus tox.** *(Rhus toxicodendron)* 6c. Use if joint pain is worst first thing in the morning or after a period of rest, then gets better with continued motion. The pain is relieved by heat but made worse by damp, cold air. One dose four times a day, for up to two weeks.

▲▲▲▲▲▲▲▲▲▲▲▲▲▲▲▲▲▲▲▲▲▲▲▲▲▲▲▲

▼▼▼▼▼▼▼▼▼▼▼▼▼▼▼▼▼▼▼▼▼▼▼▼▼▼▼

ACUPRESSURE FOR ARTHRITIS

Use one or more of the following acupressure points to ease the pain of osteoarthritis or rheumatoid arthritis. For information on acupressure, see page 29. For diagrams showing the specific pressure points, see pages 34–37.

- **Bladder 10.** One finger width below the base of the skull on the ropy muscles, a half inch outward from either side of the spine. Relieves neck and back pain.

- **Gallbladder 20.** Just below the base of the skull, in the hollow between the two large neck muscles, two to three inches apart, depending on the size of the head. Relieves arthritic pain throughout the body.

- **Large Intestine 4.** On the outside of the hand, in the webbing between the thumb and index fingers, at the highest spot of the muscle when the thumb and index fingers are brought close together. Reduces inflammation and eases arthritis pain throughout the body, especially in the hands, wrists, elbows, and shoulders.

- **Pericardium 7.** In the middle of the inside wrist crease. Relieves pain in the palms of the hands and the middle fingers.

- **Stomach 36.** Four finger widths below the kneecap and one finger width outside of the shinbone. Relieves arthritis pain throughout the body, especially in the knees.

- **Triple Warmer 4.** Follow the outside of the arm to the hollow in the center of the wrist case. Relieves wrist, forearm, and elbow pain; reduces wrist inflammation and improves wrist flexibility.

▲▲▲▲▲▲▲▲▲▲▲▲▲▲▲▲▲▲▲▲▲▲▲▲▲▲▲▲▲▲

ARTHRITIS: RHEUMATOID ARTHRITIS

Rheumatoid arthritis is an immune-system disorder in which the body turns on itself and attacks the joints and organs. The illness actually affects the entire body, causing joint inflammation, as well as inflammation of the muscles, blood vessels, skin, and sometimes even the heart and lungs. The illness damages the membranes that surround the joint-lubricating fluids, causing them to become inflamed and thickened. Affected joints deteriorate, becoming unstable, painful, swollen, and greatly misshapen. The onset occurs in children and before age forty in adults. Stress, poor nutrition, and bacterial infections can be onset factors.

In some cases, a person experiences a single bout with the illness (monocyclic rheumatoid arthritis); other times the illness alternates between an active and dormant state (polycyclic rheumatoid arthritis). However, in most cases, the disease results in chronic ongoing pain and treatment.

R̲ₓ for Health

Nutritional Supplements

Take these supplements daily for six weeks. Then take them five days, with weekends off, as a maintenance dose.

- **Take 1.8 grams of fish oil (EPA or eicosapentaenoic acid) daily.** These polyunsaturated fatty acids have been shown to relieve inflammation and the symptoms of rheumatoid arthritis.

- **Take 1500 milligrams of vitamin C and 800 IU of vitamin E daily.** Both of these vitamins are powerful antioxidants, which help prevent damage to cartilage in the joints. Vitamin C also helps with the manufacture of collagen, a protein in cartilage; without enough vitamin C, the body stops producing collagen and the joints become compromised.

- **Take up to 45 milligrams of zinc daily.** People suffering from rheumatoid arthritis often have low blood levels of zinc.

Diet

- **Eat 1 or 2 half-cup servings of flavonoid-rich foods daily.** The pigments that give fruits and flowers their color are known as flavonoids. In the body, flavonoids have anti-inflammatory and antiviral properties. The flavonoids in blueberries, cherries, grapes, and blackberries support the formation of collagen.

ASTHMA

Asthma involves recurring episodes of wheezing and breathlessness characterized by a tightening of the chest. During an attack, breathing out is obstructed, caused by spasms in the muscle surrounding the bronchi and bronchioles (the lung airway tubes). Symptoms include choking sensations, chest tightness, rapid breathing, and coughing with increased mucus secretion. Attacks most often occur at night, during exercise, or at times of emotional stress.

Allergies trigger many asthma attacks, especially allergies to pollen, animal dander, or tobacco smoke. For some people, asthma attacks are relatively mild; for others they can be life-threatening and require emergency medical treatment.

R̢ for Health

Nutritional Supplements

Take these supplements daily for two months. After that time, take them as needed, when symptoms arise.

- **Take 50 milligrams of B-complex vitamins.** The B-complex vitamins have been found to reduce both the frequency and severity of asthma attacks.

- **Take 1500 milligrams of magnesium and 750 milligrams of calcium daily.** Deficiencies in these minerals have been found to cause some attacks. The magnesium helps relax the smooth muscles of the airways, which allows them to open up.

- **Take 1500 milligrams of vitamin C daily.** People with asthma have been found to have significantly lower levels of vitamin C in the blood; studies have shown that vitamin C helps prevent bronchial spasms.

- **Take 400 IU of vitamin E daily.** This antioxidant helps reduce inflammation in the airways.

Herbal Remedies

Use these herbs daily for two months. After that time, take them as needed, when symptoms arise.

- **Take lobelia and capsicum during asthma attacks.** The herbs lobelia (*Lobelia inflata*) and capsicum (red pepper) can be helpful in controlling asthma attacks once they are under way. Keep on hand a mixture of 3 parts tincture of lobelia with 1 part tincture of capsicum. (Both tinctures should be available at a health food store.) At the start of an asthma attack, drink a small glass of water containing 20 drops of the tincture mixture. Repeat every 30 minutes for up to 3 doses. NOTE: This treatment should not replace medication prescribed by your doctor. Discuss the use of these herbs as a supplement to your conventional treatment with your physician.

- **Take 250 milligrams of licorice root three times a day.** This herb has anti-inflammatory and antiallergy properties. It also helps to prevent some of the side effects associated with the use of cortisone, one of the drugs sometimes used to treat asthma.

CATARACTS

Cataracts afflict most people over age sixty, but evidence suggests that this eye disease is preventable—and even reversible in early stages. Poor nutrition, especially a diet high in sugar, fat, and white flour, is a major cause of cataracts.

Cataracts occur when the crystalline lens of the eye grows cloudy or opaque. Cataracts form when the eye loses the ability to maintain appropriate concentrations of sodium, potassium, and calcium within the lens. In many cases, the mineral imbalance in the lens stems from damage caused by free radicals due to exposure to ultraviolet light or low-level radiation from X rays. Cataracts can also be caused by disease, particularly diabetes, eye injury, use of certain steroids, and a congenital defect.

Regular eye exams are essential to identify cataracts in the early stages, since special equipment is required to identify them (the classic white film doesn't appear over the eyes until the cataracts are quite advanced).

R̥ for Health

Nutritional Supplements

Use one or more of the following nutritional supplements five days, with weekends off, on an ongoing basis.

- **Take a B-complex vitamin containing 10 milligrams of riboflavin (vitamin B₂).** Cataracts have been linked to a deficiency in riboflavin, a B vitamin that helps with metabolism. (About one out of every three people over age sixty-five is riboflavin deficient.) Taking a B-complex vitamin keeps the various B vitamins in balance.

- **Take 1000 milligrams of vitamin C daily, in divided doses.** Studies show that vitamin C lowers pressure in the eye and helps halt the progression of cataracts. It also protects the lens of the eye because it is a free-radical scavenger. One study found that people who took between 300 and 600 milligrams of vitamin C had a 70-percent reduction in cataract risk. Protective effects appear with the intake of as little as 120 milligrams, the equivalent of 1 cup of orange juice or ½ cup of strawberries.

- **Take 800 IU of vitamin E and 50 micrograms of selenium daily.** These free-radical destroyers work together to protect the eyes. A selenium deficiency has been linked to the formation of cataracts; in fact, the selenium content in lenses with cataracts is only 15 percent of the level found in healthy eyes.

Herbal Remedies

- **Take 100 milligrams of bilberry extract daily.** Bilberry, the European version of blueberry, has long been used to treat eye problems. Bilberry contains bioflavonoids called anthocyanins, which improve circulation to the blood vessels of the eye. (Blueberries also contain anthocyanins, but there are higher concentrations in bilberry.)

▼▼▼▼▼▼▼▼▼▼▼▼▼▼▼▼▼▼▼▼▼▼▼▼▼▼▼▼

Preventive Care

To reduce your risk of developing cataracts, wear sunglasses and a wide-brimmed hat when outdoors in bright sunlight. Eat a diet rich in antioxidants to minimize the risk of free-radical damage to the eyes.

▲▲▲▲▲▲▲▲▲▲▲▲▲▲▲▲▲▲▲▲▲▲▲▲▲▲▲▲

▼▼▼▼▼▼▼▼▼▼▼▼▼▼▼▼▼▼▼▼▼▼▼▼▼▼▼▼

Homeopathy for Cataracts

Use one homeopathic treatment at a time, based on your specific symptoms. For information on homeopathy, see page 23. Discontinue use if the symptoms disappear.

- **Calcarea** (*Calcarea carbonica*) 6c. Use in the early stages of cataract formation. One dose three times a day, for up to seven days. If your condition improves, take one dose twice a day for two weeks more. If your condition does not improve, contact a homeopath or another health professional.

- **Silicea** (*Silicea terra*) 6c. Use in later stages of the disease, when the cataract interferes with sight. One dose three times a day, for up to seven days. If your condition improves, take one dose twice a day for two weeks more. If your condition does not improve, contact a homeopath or another health professional.

▲▲▲▲▲▲▲▲▲▲▲▲▲▲▲▲▲▲▲▲▲▲▲▲▲▲▲▲

▼▼▼▼▼▼▼▼▼▼▼▼▼▼▼▼▼▼▼▼▼▼▼▼

ACUPRESSURE FOR CATARACTS

Use one or more of the following acupressure points. For information on acupressure, see page 29. For a diagram showing the specific pressure points, see pages 34–37.

- **Gallbladder 1.** In the slight depression level with the outside corner of the eye.

- **Stomach 1.** Directly below the pupil of the eye, in the center of the ridge of the bony socket below the eye.

- **Stomach 8.** At the corner of the forehead, one finger width inside the hairline.

- **Triple Warmer 23.** In the slight depression at the outer edge of the eyebrow.

▲▲▲▲▲▲▲▲▲▲▲▲▲▲▲▲▲▲▲▲▲▲▲▲

CONSTIPATION

As anyone who has ever experienced it already knows, constipation involves straining to pass hard, dry stools; it can also include gas pains and bloating. In severe cases, it can cause the digestive system to halt completely, resulting in an impacted bowel.

Constipation is not defined by frequency of bowel movements, since there is no single definition of the "normal" number of bowel movements a person should have each day. In general, the body eliminates waste in eighteen to twenty-four hours with a high-fiber diet or forty-eight hours with a low-fiber diet.

Constipation can be caused by a poor diet containing too little fiber and too much refined flour, sugar, meat, and dairy products. Lack of exercise, liver or gallbladder disease, stress and anxiety, hypothyroidism, anemia, food allergies, and not drinking enough water are also contributing factors. Too frequent use of laxatives or enemas can make bowel action lazy and result in chronic constipation or laxative dependency. The straining associated with constipation can result in more serious problems, such as diverticulitis, hemorrhoids, hernias, and varicose veins.

R̷ for Health

Diet
The following dietary recommendations can be used on an ongoing basis for overall health:

- **Eat a high-fiber diet.** Eating a diet rich in high-fiber foods—such as fruits, vegetables, whole wheat bread, and bran—can ease constipation. Water-insoluble fibers such as cellulose tend to increase stool weight by attracting and holding water. Be sure to increase your fluid intake when you increase your dietary fiber.

- **Drink at least eight 8-ounce glasses of water every day.** Water is essential for keeping stools soft. Keep in mind that alcoholic and caffeinated beverages do not contribute to your daily requirements.

- **Eat one or two apples a day.** Apples are high in fiber, which help encourage bowel movements. You can also take 500 milligrams of apple pectin in supplement form until the constipation has passed.

Nutritional Supplements
The following supplements can be used for three or four days to help you overcome an episode of constipation. If constipation persists, see your physician or health care practitioner to find out what is causing the problem.

- **Take 1 to 2 rounded teaspoons of psyllium seeds after each meal in a full glass of water.** These seeds, sometimes referred to as Mother Nature's laxative, are the active ingredient in many over-the-counter laxative preparations.

- **Take 400 to 800 IU of vitamin E daily.** This vitamin helps to heal an irritated colon.

- **Take 1 teaspoon of *Lactobacillus acidophilus* daily.** This supplement boosts the levels of beneficial bacteria in the intestine, which can help with digestion and relieve constipation.

▼▼▼▼▼▼▼▼▼▼▼▼▼▼▼▼▼▼▼▼▼▼▼▼▼▼▼

HOMEOPATHY FOR CONSTIPATION

Use one homeopathic treatment at a time, based on your specific symptoms. For information on homeopathy, see page 23. Discontinue use if the symptoms disappear.

- **Alumina** *(Alumina)* 6c. Use when even soft stools are difficult to pass; they may be mucus-covered or claylike. One dose every two hours, for up to ten doses.

- **Bryonia** *(Bryonia alba)* 30c. Use when the stools are large, dry, and hard. One dose every two hours, for up to ten doses.

- **Nux** *(Strychnos nux vomica)* 6c. Use when there is an urge to eliminate but little or no success in passing stools; often there is a feeling that there is more to come. One dose every two hours, for up to ten doses.

- **Silicea** *(Silicea terra)* 6c. Use when the stool passes the anal sphincter, then slips back again; stools tend to be hard and mucus-covered. One dose every two hours, for up to ten doses.

▲▲▲▲▲▲▲▲▲▲▲▲▲▲▲▲▲▲▲▲▲▲▲▲▲▲▲

▼▼▼▼▼▼▼▼▼▼▼▼▼▼▼▼▼▼▼▼▼▼▼▼▼▼▼

ACUPRESSURE FOR CONSTIPATION

Use one or more of the following acupressure points. For information on acupressure, see page 29. For diagrams showing the specific pressure points, see pages 34–36.

- **Bladder 25.** Two finger widths on either side of the spinal column, level with the top of the hipbones.

- **Conception Vessel 6.** Two to three finger widths below the belly button.

- **Large Intestine 4.** At the end of the crease made by the index finger and thumb when they are pressed together.

- **Large Intestine 11.** In the depression at the end of the elbow crease, when the elbow is slightly bent.

- **Spleen 8.** On the inside of the lower leg, four finger widths below the knee, in the depression under the bone.

- **Stomach 34.** Three finger widths above the kneecap, in the depression on the outer edge of the muscle.

▲▲▲▲▲▲▲▲▲▲▲▲▲▲▲▲▲▲▲▲▲▲▲▲▲▲

DEPRESSION

At some point in their lives, most people experience depression. People often confuse sadness and depression. While we all feel sadness in response to certain situations, depression is characterized by ongoing feelings of worthlessness, pessimism, sadness, and apathy toward life. With clinical depression, these feelings linger for weeks or months and can become incapacitating.

Some people inherit a tendency to develop depression due to their brain chemistry. Other times the illness is brought on by physical conditions, such as stroke, chronic stress, thyroid disease, menopause, alcoholism, drug abuse, hepatitis, or the lack of sunlight during winter months. Some drugs, including over-the-counter antihistamines and many prescription drugs, can trigger depression as well. Severe depression can be life-threatening. If your depression seems overwhelming or if it persists even after trying the following remedies for several weeks, seek professional help. Consider discussing the issue with your primary care physician, who can then make a referral to an appropriate mental health professional.

R~x~ for Health

The following supplements and herbs can be used on an ongoing basis.
Take supplements five days, then take the weekends off. Discontinue
use for several weeks in the spring and summer and see if the depression returns. If these supplements are not helpful in easing the symptoms of depression, seek care from your physician or a mental health
professional.

Nutritional Supplements

- **Take 1500 milligrams of magnesium and 750 milligrams of
  calcium daily.** Studies have shown that people who experience
  depression often have low levels of these minerals.

- **Take up to 3000 milligrams of vitamin C daily, in divided
  doses.** This antioxidant vitamin is necessary for the synthesis of
  neurotransmitters in the brain. It can help ease the symptoms of
  depression.

- **Take 500 milligrams of 5-HTP.** This chemical is the precursor to
  serotonin in the brain. 5-HTP can be found in some health food
  stores or from some health care professionals. Follow package
  directions.

Herbal Remedies

- **Take 300 milligrams of Saint-John's-wort three times a day.**
  This herb has long been used as a mood enhancer and antidepressant. It contains hypericum, a chemical that blocks the action of
  monoamine oxidase in the body. (MAO inhibitors are a common
  class of prescription antidepressant drugs.) Look for capsules containing .3 percent hypericum. NOTE: While taking this herb, do
  not take amphetamines, narcotics, diet pills, asthma inhalants,
  decongestants, or cold or hay fever medication.

Diet

- **Use basil liberally in cooking.** This herb has antidepressant
  properties. Also consider adding five drops of essential oil of basil
  to bathwater for a soothing and uplifting bath.

- **Eat plenty of oatmeal.** Oatmeal and oat products have antidepressant and mood-elevating properties. Eat oatmeal or use a commercially prepared oat extract.

▼▼▼▼▼▼▼▼▼▼▼▼▼▼▼▼▼▼▼▼▼▼▼▼▼▼

PREVENTIVE CARE

We all feel sad from time to time, but we don't all become clinically depressed. Severe or ongoing depression may be treated by a mental health professional. You may prevent some types of depression by getting regular exercise and rest, and by talking to someone about your feelings.

▲▲▲▲▲▲▲▲▲▲▲▲▲▲▲▲▲▲▲▲▲▲▲▲▲▲

▼▼▼▼▼▼▼▼▼▼▼▼▼▼▼▼▼▼▼▼▼▼▼▼▼▼

HOMEOPATHY FOR DEPRESSION

Use one homeopathic treatment at a time, based on your specific symptoms. For information on homeopathy, see page 23. Discontinue use if the symptoms disappear.

- **Aurum** (*Aurum metallicum*) 6c. Use when suicidal feelings and self-loathing accompany depression. One dose three times a day, for two weeks. NOTE: If someone feels suicidal, seek professional help or call a suicide hotline in addition to using natural remedies.

- **Ignatia** (*Ignatia amara*) 6c. Use when depression follows a heartbreak or deep grief and is accompanied by mood swings; behavior may be inappropriate for a given situation. One dose three times a day, for up to two weeks.

- **Nux** (*Strychnos nux vomica*) 6c. Use when depression is accompanied by irritability. One dose three times a day, for two weeks.

- **Pulsatilla** *(Pulsatilla nigricans)* 6c. Use when tearfulness and self-pity accompany depression. One dose three times a day, for up to two weeks.

▲▲▲▲▲▲▲▲▲▲▲▲▲▲▲▲▲▲▲▲▲▲▲▲▲▲▲▲▲▲

▼▼▼▼▼▼▼▼▼▼▼▼▼▼▼▼▼▼▼▼▼▼▼▼▼▼▼▼▼▼

ACUPRESSURE FOR DEPRESSION

Use one or more of the following acupressure points. For information on acupressure, see page 29. For diagrams showing the specific pressure points, see pages 34–35.

- **Bladder 10.** Just inside the hairline on the nape of the neck, a half inch out on either side of the spine, in the depression on the side of the large neck muscles.

- **Conception Vessel 12.** Along the center of the abdomen, halfway between the navel and the edge of the breastbone.

- **Governing Vessel 26.** Halfway up the groove below the nose. NOTE: Avoid using this pressure point if you have high blood pressure.

- **Liver 3.** On the top of the foot, in the web between the first and second toes.

▲▲▲▲▲▲▲▲▲▲▲▲▲▲▲▲▲▲▲▲▲▲▲▲▲▲▲▲▲▲

HEMORRHOIDS

Four out of five Americans experience hemorrhoids at some point in their lives, but few people want to talk about them. Hemorrhoids, those inflamed and widened veins that look like purple skin growths around the anus, can be painful, itchy, and quite uncomfortable.

Hemorrhoids (also known as piles) can appear either outside or inside the anus. They can be caused by constipation, obesity, pregnancy, improper diet, lack of exercise, heavy weight lifting, or liver damage. The condition tends to run in families.

R̥ for Health

Diet

- **Eat a high-fiber diet.** Few of our African ancestors experienced hemorrhoids, which are rare in cultures where people eat a high-fiber diet. Eat plenty of whole grains and fresh fruits and vegetables.

- **Eat blackberries, cherries, and blueberries.** These fruits contain chemicals (proanthocyanidin and anthocyanidin) that help to strengthen the veins. To assist in the treatment of hemorrhoids, be sure to include these fruits in your daily diet.

Herbal Remedies

The following herbal remedies can be used for up to one week. If symptoms persist after that time, consult a doctor or medical professional.

- **Apply a witch hazel compress.** Used topically, witch hazel can help shrink blood vessels and stop minor bleeding. A witch hazel tincture or concentrated herbal drops are preferable to witch hazel liniments containing methyl or wood alcohol; witch hazel products can be found in health food stores and conventional pharmacies. For extra relief, chill the witch hazel in the refrigerator before using.

- **Take 100 milligrams of butcher's broom three times a day.** This herb helps to strengthen the veins in the rectum.

- **Take 1 capsule of stoneroot daily.** This herb works exceptionally well on hemorrhoids, strengthening the veins and acting as an astringent. Powders and tinctures are commercially available from health food stores; follow package directions.

▼▼▼▼▼▼▼▼▼▼▼▼▼▼▼▼▼▼▼▼▼▼▼▼

HOMEOPATHY FOR HEMORRHOIDS

Use one homeopathic treatment at a time, based on your specific symptoms. For information on homeopathy, see page 23. Discontinue use if the symptoms disappear.

- **Aesculus** (*Aesculus hippocastanum*) 6c. Use when hemorrhoids accompany constipation and the stools are lumpy. One dose four times a day, for up to five days.

- **Capsicum** (*Capsicum annum*) 6c. Use when hemorrhoids protrude from the anus and burn. One dose four times a day, for up to five days.

- **Hamamelis** (*Hamamelis virginiana*). Use when hemorrhoids bleed or feel strained. One dose four times a day, for up to five days.

- **Nitric ac.** (*Nitricum acidum*) 6c. Use when anal fissures accompany hemorrhoids and there is pain before, during, and after bowel movements. One dose four times a day, for up to five days.

▲▲▲▲▲▲▲▲▲▲▲▲▲▲▲▲▲▲▲▲▲▲▲▲

▼▼▼▼▼▼▼▼▼▼▼▼▼▼▼▼▼▼▼▼▼▼▼▼

ACUPRESSURE FOR HEMORRHOIDS

Use one or more of the following acupressure points. For information on acupressure, see page 29. For diagrams showing the specific pressure points, see pages 35–36.

- **Large Intestine 4.** On the outside of the hand, in the webbing between the thumb and index finger. The point is located at the highest spot of muscle when the thumb and index finger are brought together.

- **Large Intestine 11.** On the arm, at the outer edge of the elbow crease.

- **Stomach 36.** Four finger widths below the kneecap and one finger width outside the shinbone. (If you're in the right spot, you'll be able to feel your muscle flex as you move your foot up and down.)

▲▲▲▲▲▲▲▲▲▲▲▲▲▲▲▲▲▲▲▲▲▲▲▲▲▲▲▲▲▲▲

IMPOTENCE

Sooner or later, it happens to almost *every* man. Still, most of our male patients feel very embarrassed when we talk about impotence, a chronic problem achieving and maintaining an erection long enough to experience intercourse. We try to assure those patients that they are not alone—an estimated ten to twenty million American men are chronically impotent—but too often these men feel that their sexual identity is linked to their sexual performance.

Roughly three-fourths of all erection problems have at least some physical cause. To achieve an erection there must be cooperation of blood vessels, nerves, and tissues. A number of health problems—including diabetes, heart and circulation problems, stroke, epilepsy, Alzheimer's disease, neurological disorders, alcohol and drug abuse, Parkinson's disease, and liver and kidney disease—can cause impotence. So can certain medications, including tranquilizers, diuretics, and anti-ulcer, antipsychotic, antidepressant, and antihypertensive drugs. Some over-the-counter antihistamines and decongestants can also cause temporary impotence.

The other causes of impotence stem from psychological factors. With patience and treatment, most cases of psychological—as well as physical—impotence can be managed and overcome.

R̲x for Health

Nutritional Supplements

Take the following nutritional supplements five days a week on an ongoing basis:

- **Take 15 milligrams of zinc daily.** A man's prostate gland function and overall reproductive health depends on the adequate intake of zinc.

- **Take 50 milligrams of niacin (vitamin B$_3$) daily.** This vasodilator increases the blood flow throughout the body, including the penis.

- **Take a multiple vitamin/mineral supplement containing at least 5000 IU of vitamin A every day.** The body needs vitamin A to produce the sex hormones that are essential for sexual function. Eat orange vegetables and other foods rich in beta-carotene (which the body converts to vitamin A). A good multiple vitamin/mineral supplement should provide an adequate amount of this important vitamin.

Herbal Remedies

The following herbs can be used as a tonic for overall health. Use them for six weeks. If you notice an improvement in your condition, continue to use them five days a week, taking weekends off.

- **Under a doctor's supervision, use a commercial herbal preparation containing yohimbe.** This herb is the primary ingredient in a prescription drug used to treat impotency by increasing blood flow. It is commercially available, often in so-called male potency formulas. Follow package directions.

- **Use a commercial herbal preparation containing ginseng.** This herb has long been considered a mild aphrodisiac. Ginseng preparations are widely available in health food stores; follow package directions.

- **Use a commercial herbal product containing ginkgo.** This herb helps improve blood flow to the penis, which can help combat impotence. Ginkgo is usually available only as a commercial preparation; follow package directions.

MEDICAL TESTS FOR IMPOTENCE

When a patient complains of impotence, the first thing we do is take steps to rule out a physical cause of the problem. This is usually done by a series of tests to assess the blood flow to the penis, the condition of the spinal cord, and testosterone and blood glucose levels. In some cases, we recommend an at-home sleep test to find out if a man experiences erections during sleep (if you have no erections during sleep, then there is probably a physical cause for the problem; if you do experience erections at night but not when you are with a partner, the problem probably has psychological origins).

If tests reveal that a man's hormone levels fall below normal levels, we may prescribe testosterone shots, skin patches, or supplements. In rare cases, if there is inadequate blood flow to the penis, surgery may be required to open or unblock the arteries to the penis. And, if all else fails, we may suggest a man consider erection-producing medications or assistive devices.

SEXY FOODS

Many foods traditionally believed to improve sexual function come from the ocean. Fish and shellfish (particularly oysters and clams) are thought to be good for sexual function, perhaps due to their high levels of zinc. Seaweeds, which provide a rich source of minerals, also come from the ocean and support sexual function. On the other hand, milk and milk products, such as cheese and ice cream, can have a sedative effect on sexual energy. So if you're interested in a night of romance, enjoy a seafood dinner, but pass on the ice cream for dessert.

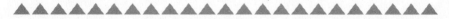

HOMEOPATHY FOR IMPOTENCE

Use one homeopathic treatment at a time, based on your specific symptoms. For information on homeopathy, see page 23. Discontinue use if the symptoms disappear.

- **Agnus** *(Agnus castus)* 30c. Use when intercourse has been frequent but the erection is suddenly not firm enough for penetration. One dose twice daily, for up to five days.

- **Conium** *(Conium maculatum)* 30c. Use when there has been a long period without intercourse and there is desire but the erection does not last. One dose twice daily, for up to five days.

- **Ignatia** *(Ignatia amara)* 30c. Use when distracted by grief or stress in other relationships. One dose twice daily, for up to five days.

- **Lycopodium** *(Lycopodium clavatum)* 30c. Use when the man would like to have intercourse but fears failure. One dose twice daily, for up to five days.

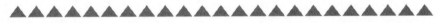

ACUPRESSURE FOR IMPOTENCE

Use one or more of the following acupressure points. For information on acupressure, see page 29. For diagrams showing the specific pressure points, see pages 34–37.

- **Bladder 23.** Two finger widths away from the spine at waist level (in line with the belly button).

- **Conception Vessel 6.** Three finger widths below the belly button.

- **Kidney 1.** At the base of the ball of the foot, in the middle of the sole.

- **Kidney 3.** Inside the ankle, in the depression between the back of the ankle and the Achilles tendon.

- **Spleen 12.** In the center of the crease where the leg joins the trunk.

▲▲▲▲▲▲▲▲▲▲▲▲▲▲▲▲▲▲▲▲▲▲▲▲▲▲▲▲▲

INSOMNIA

Insomnia is a real nightmare: You desperately want to sleep, but it seems impossible to doze off. Insomnia refers to any of three sleep disorders: difficulty falling asleep (more than forty-five minutes), early morning awakening, or frequent night awakenings (six or more a night). You have insomnia if any of these symptoms leave you feeling tired and worn down in the morning.

Most people have trouble sleeping from time to time. In fact, during the course of a year, nearly one out of every three people suffers from insomnia at least once. Short-term insomnia (from a few nights to a few weeks) usually stems from worry or stress. Long-term insomnia (from a few months to a few years) often comes from general anxiety, depression, chronic pain, hypoglycemia, apnea, or a side effect of a medication you may be taking.

R̞ for Health
Nutritional Supplements
Use the following supplements five days a week on an ongoing basis.

- **Take 1000 milligrams of calcium and 1000 milligrams of magnesium daily.** A deficiency in calcium and magnesium can cause you to wake up after a few hours of sleep and have trouble getting back to sleep.

Diet

The following dietary changes can be used as long as needed.

- **Eat foods high in tryptophan before heading to bed.** Before turning in, snack on foods high in sleep-producing tryptophan, such as whole grain crackers, peanut butter, figs, dates, tuna, turkey, bananas, yogurt, and milk, if necessary.

- **Avoid foods containing tyramines before trying to sleep.** Foods that contain tyramines cause the brain to release norepinephrine, a natural stimulant. In the evening before bed, pass on tyramine-rich foods, such as caffeine, alcohol, sugar, tobacco, cheese, chocolate, sauerkraut, wine, bacon, ham, sausage, eggplant, potatoes, spinach, and tomatoes.

Herbal Remedies

The following herbs can be used for up to six weeks. If they seem helpful, continue using them five days a week, with weekends off.

- **Take 300 milligrams of valerian forty-five minutes before bedtime.** This herb has been widely used in folk medicine as a sedative; clinical studies have also demonsrated the sleep-enhancing benefits of valerian.

- **Take 300 milligrams of passionflower forty-five minutes before bedtime.** This herb was used as a sedative by the Aztecs; it can be helpful in promoting rest.

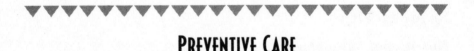

PREVENTIVE CARE

To prevent insomnia, get regular exercise, but avoid strenuous exercise two hours before bedtime.

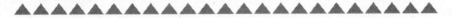

▼▼▼▼▼▼▼▼▼▼▼▼▼▼▼▼▼▼▼▼▼▼▼▼

HOMEOPATHY FOR INSOMNIA

Use one homeopathic treatment at a time, based on your specific symptoms. For information on homeopathy, see page 23. Discontinue use if the symptoms disappear.

- **Aconite** (*Aconitum napellus*) 30c. Use if nightmares, particularly about death, accompany sleep problems. One dose one hour before bed, for one week. Repeat if you wake up and can't get back to sleep.

- **Coffea** (*Coffea cruda*) 30c. Use if your mind is active and you toss and turn all night. One dose one hour before bed, for one week. Repeat if you wake up and can't get back to sleep.

- **Ignatia** (*Ignatia amara*) 30c. Use if you are fearful of bedtime, possibly due to nightmares. One dose one hour before bed, for one week. Repeat if you wake up and can't get back to sleep.

- **Nux** (*Strychnos nux vomica*) 30c. Use if you fall asleep but wake up at 3 A.M. or so and remain awake, perhaps falling asleep again just before morning. One dose one hour before bed, for one week. Repeat if you wake up with nightmares and can't get back to sleep.

▲▲▲▲▲▲▲▲▲▲▲▲▲▲▲▲▲▲▲▲▲▲▲▲▲

▼▼▼▼▼▼▼▼▼▼▼▼▼▼▼▼▼▼▼▼▼▼▼▼

ACUPRESSURE FOR INSOMNIA

Use one or more of the following acupressure points. For information on acupressure, see page 29. For diagrams showing the specific pressure points, see pages 36–37.

- **Bladder 62.** In the first indentation directly below the outer anklebone.

- **Gallbladder 12.** Behind the ears, in the hollow under the bone.

- **Heart 7.** On the inside of the wrist crease, in the hollow level with the little finger.

- **Kidney 6.** Directly below the inside of the anklebone, in a slight indentation.

▲▲▲▲▲▲▲▲▲▲▲▲▲▲▲▲▲▲▲▲▲▲▲▲▲▲▲▲

MIGRAINE HEADACHES

A migraine is no simple headache. The throbbing pain can be completely incapacitating. The pain usually begins with an intense, throbbing pain, which spreads. Some people also experience nausea and vomiting. Migraines can last from several hours to several days. In most cases, the headache peaks within an hour, lasts four to twenty-four hours, and happens several times a month.

About half of all people experience a warning sign—such as blurred vision, bright spots in the vision, muddled thinking, numbness, or tingling—before the pain begins. During a migraine, many people experience sensitivity to light, odors, and sound. Migraines seem to be linked to changes in the blood vessels in the head; the disorder may be caused by an imbalance in the brain chemical serotonin.

℞ for Health

Nutritional Supplements
Use the following supplement five days a week on an ongoing basis.

- **Take 200 milligrams of magnesium three times a day.** Magnesium relaxes constricted blood vessels; taking supplemental magnesium can help prevent some migraine headaches.

Diet

- **Avoid foods that can trigger migraines.** A number of foods have been associated with migraine headaches, including alcohol, chocolate, aged cheese, processed meats, shellfish, monosodium glutamate (MSG), red wine, and citrus fruits. Consider keeping a food diary to document the foods you eat prior to your migraine attacks.

Herbal Remedies

- **Take 125 milligrams of feverfew daily.** This is the most commonly used herb for the prevention and treatment of migraine headaches. It is thought to work by blocking excessive secretion of serotonin, a neurotransmitter in the brain. A single daily dose can be helpful in preventing headaches. To manage the pain after an acute attack, take three capsules at once, then again every four hours. Don't exceed twelve capsules in a day.

SKIN PROBLEMS

African Americans face special skin care issues. Our dark skin tends to be firmer and smoother than white skin; however, African Americans experience several skin problems, including:

- Acne. This is a condition in which the sebaceous glands become blocked with oil and dead skin, allowing bacteria to grow and pimples to form.

- Eczema. Skin with eczema becomes itchy, red, scaly, or peeling, often in response to an environmental irritant, such as metals, perfumes, cosmetics, rubber, plants, and certain medications. Stress, asthma, hay fever, and allergies can also trigger eczema.

- Hyperpigmentation. This condition involves the formation of dark patches of skin that can take months to fade; the condition is usually caused by acne, insect bites, hair bumps, or some other source of irritation.

- Keloids. These are raised scars caused by the overhealing of a cut, scrape, burn, or break in the skin; the tendency to develop keloids often runs in families.

- Vitiligo. This skin disease involves the loss of skin pigment, usually starting with the fingers, feet, and around the mouth and eyes; the cause is unknown.

While some skin problems are best treated by a dermatologist, the following remedies can be helpful in managing simple skin outbreaks.

R̥ for Health

Nutritional Supplements
Use the following supplement daily for six weeks. If it proves helpful, continue to use it on an ongoing basis. Take it five days, then take the weekends off.

- **Take 1 teaspoon of flaxseed oil three times daily.** The essential fatty acids are vital for healing skin diseases, especially acne, eczema, and dermatitis. The oil can also be applied topically. Other fatty acids that can be substituted include salmon oil, cod liver oil, black currant oil, sesame seed oil, and linseed oil.

Herbal Remedies
Use the following herbs daily for six weeks. If they prove helpful, continue to use them on an ongoing basis. Take them five days, then take the weekends off.

- **Drink up to 3 cups of basil tea daily.** Basil kills bacteria on the skin. Prepare an infusion of basil by adding 3 teaspoons of dried basil leaves to 1 cup of boiling water. Steep for 10 to 15 minutes, strain, and enjoy.

- **Wash with calendula soap.** Calendula soap soothes irritated skin and helps fight infection. Wash with this herbal soap (available at health food stores) and be sure to rinse thoroughly with lukewarm water.

- **Take 250 milligrams of licorice daily.** This herb helps to reduce the histamine production common in people with skin disorders. It helps fight inflammation and irritation.

- **Take 500 milligrams of burdock.** This herb is quite effective in the treatment of eczema. It strengthens the immune system and helps control the bacterial infections that can cause eczema.

VARICOSE VEINS

If you have varicose veins, blame them on gravity. The blood that circulates to the legs must be pumped uphill to the heart, against the pull of gravity. Veins are equipped with one-way valves to prevent the blood from flowing back down the legs, but when the valves are stretched or damaged, they don't close properly, and the blood slips back down and pools, causing the veins to stretch out and appear puffy and discolored.

Pregnancy and childbirth weaken the valves in the veins and contribute to the problem, as does standing for long periods of time or sitting with crossed legs. Genetics and obesity also play a role. In most cases, varicose veins don't pose a health problem. However, those that form deep within the leg should be treated by a medical professional, since they can lead to skin ulcers, phlebitis (inflammation of the vein), and thrombosis (a blood clot).

℞ for Health

Nutritional Supplements
The following supplement can be used on an ongoing basis.

- **Take 400 to 800 IU of vitamin E daily.** This antioxidant vitamin helps improve circulation and prevent a heavy feeling in the legs.

Diet
- **Eat 3 servings of flavonoid-rich berries a day.** Cherries, blueberries, blackberries, and other flavonoid-rich berries help prevent

and treat varicose veins by strengthening the walls of the veins. Eat these richly colored berries every day.

- **Eat a high-fiber diet.** Varicose veins may be exacerbated by a low-fiber diet, which can result in straining during a bowel movement. Over time the straining may weaken the vein walls, resulting in both varicose veins and hemorrhoids.

Herbal Remedies

The following herbal remedies can be used five days a week on an on-going basis.

- **Take 60 to 120 milligrams of gotu kola extract daily.** Clinical studies have shown that gotu kola extract helps improve varicose veins, probably because it enhances connective tissue structure and improves blood flow. For an infusion, use ½ teaspoon of dried herb per cup of boiling water. Strain and drink up to 2 cups a day. Commercially prepared tinctures are also available; follow package directions.

- **Take 100 milligrams of butcher's broom three times daily.** This herb contains ruscogenins, compounds known to fight inflammation and constrict the veins.

- **Apply a compress of horse chestnut 15 minutes three or four times a day during periods of acute discomfort.** This herb fights inflammation, decreases the number and size of the small pores of the capillary walls, and tones the walls of the veins by strengthening their elastic fibers. A commercially prepared tincture can be taken internally (following package directions); it can also be diluted with one part water and used as a topical compress.

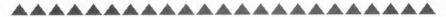

ACUPRESSURE FOR VARICOSE VEINS

Use one or more of the following acupressure points. For information on acupressure, see page 29. For diagrams showing the specific pressure points, see pages 34 and 36.

- **Kidney 6.** One thumb width below the inside of the anklebone.

- **Spleen 6.** On the inside of the leg, four finger widths above the tip of the anklebone and just inside the bone of the leg.

- **Spleen 9.** On the inside of the leg, below the knee and under the large bulge of bone.

- **Spleen 10.** On the inside edge of the top of the knee, where the opposite thumb touches the muscles when the knee is flexed.

Appendix A
Recommended Reading

ON NUTRITION

Staying Healthy with Nutrition: The Complete Guide to Diet & Nutritional Medicine by Elson M. Haas, M.D. Berkeley: Celestial Arts, 1992.

ON MIND-BODY MEDICINE

Mind as Healer, Mind as Slayer by Kenneth R. Pelletier. New York: Dell, 1992.
Anatomy of the Spirit: The Seven Stages of Power and Healing by Carolyn Myss. New York: Harmony Books, 1996.
Minding the Body, Mending the Mind by Joan Borysenko. Reading, Mass.: Addison-Wesley, 1987.

ON HERBAL MEDICINE

The Complete Medicinal Herbal by Penelope Ody. London: Dorling Kindersley, 1993.
Encyclopedia of Natural Medicine by Michael Murry, N.D., and Joseph Pizzorono, N.D. Rocklin, Calif.: Prima Publishing, 1991.

ON HOMEOPATHY

Homeopathy: The Principles and Practice of Treatment by Dr. Andrew Lockie and Dr. Nicola Geddes. London: Dorling Kindersley, 1995.

ON ACUPRESSURE

Acupressure for Health by Jacqueline Young. San Francisco: Thorsons, 1994.
Acupressure's Potent Points by Michael Reed Gach. New York: Bantam Books, 1990.

ON NATURAL PROGESTERONE

What Your Doctor May Not Tell You About Menopause by John R. Lee, M.D., and Virginia Hopkins. New York: Warner Books, 1996.

Organizations of Interest

NATUROPATHIC MEDICINE

For a referral to a naturopath or a medical doctor who specializes in natural treatments, contact:

American Association of Naturopathic Physicians
601 Valley Street
Suite 105
Seattle, WA 98109
(206) 298-0125

National College of Naturopathic Medicine
11231 S.E. Market Street
Portland, OR 97216
(503) 255-4860

HERBAL MEDICINE

For more information on herbal medicine and referrals to practitioners in your area, contact:

The American Herbalists Guild
P.O. Box 1683
Soquel, CA 95073
(408) 464-2441
(408) 469-4372

American Association of Naturopathic Physicians
601 Valley Street
Suite 105
Seattle, WA 98109
(206) 298-0125

Additional publications, newsletters, and books on herbal medicine are available from:

African American Product Company/Nia
2 Executive Park Drive
New Windsor, NY 12553
(888) 313-3103

The American Foundation of Traditional Chinese Medicine
505 Beach Street
San Francisco, CA 94133
(415) 776-0502

The American Botanical Council
P.O. Box 201660
Austin, TX 78720
(512) 331-8868
(800) 373-7105

Herb Research Foundation
1007 Pearl Street
Suite 200
Boulder, CO 80302
(303) 449-2265

Institute for Traditional Medicine
2017 Southeast Hawthorne
Portland, OR 97214
(503) 233-4907

Manufacturers of herb mail-order catalogs include:

African American Product Company/Nia
2 Executive Park Drive
New Windsor, NY 12553
(888) 313-3103

Earth's Harvest
2557 N.W. Division
Gresham, OR 97030
(800) 428-3308

East Earth Trade Winds
P.O. Box 493151
Redding, CA 96049-3151
(800) 258-6878
(916) 241-6878 in California

Eclectic Institute
14385 Lusted Road
Sandy, OR 97055
(800) 332-HERB

Herb-Pharm
P.O. Box 116
William, OR 97544
(503) 846-6262

Herbs of Grace
Division of School of Natural Medicine
P.O. Box 7369
Boulder, CO 80306-7369
(303) 443-4882

Meridian Traditional Herbal Products
44 Linden Street
Brookline, MA 02146
(800) 356-6003
(617) 739-2636 in Massachusetts

McZand Herbal Inc.
P.O. Box 5312
Santa Monica, CA 90409
(310) 822-0500

Nature's Way Products, Inc.
10 Mountain Springs Parkway
Springville, UT 84663
(801) 489-1520

Windriver Herbs
P.O. Box 3876
Jackson, WY 83001
(800) 903-HERB

DIET AND NUTRITION

For information on finding a qualified nutritionist, contact:

The American Association of Nutritional Consultants
880 Canarios Court
Suite 210
Chula Vista, CA 91910-7810
(619) 482-8533

American Academy of Nutrition
3408 Sausalito Drive
Corona Del Mar, CA 92625
(800) 290-4226

American College of Nutrition
722 Robert E. Lee Drive
Wilmington, NC 28412
(919) 452-1222

The Consumer Nutrition Hotline
(sponsored by the American Dietetic Association)
(800) 366-1655
The hotline staff can answer questions and provide free referrals
to registered dietitians in your area.

Publications on nutrition (some for a fee) are available from:

American Institute of Nutrition
9650 Rockville Pike
Suite L4500
Bethesda, MD 20814-3990
(301) 530-7050

American Council on Science and Health
1995 Broadway, 16th floor
New York, NY 10023-5860
(212) 362-7044

The Nutrition Action Health Letter
Center for Science in the Public Interest
1875 Connecticut Avenue, N.W.
Suite 300
Washington, DC 20009-5728
(202) 332-9111

Society for Nutrition Education
2001 Killebrew Drive
Suite 340
Minneapolis, MN 55425-1882
(612) 854-0035

Vegetarian Resource Group
P.O. Box 1463
Baltimore, MD 21203
(410) 366-8343

HOMEOPATHY

For an information packet on homeopathy and a directory of practitioners, contact:

The National Center for Homeopathy
801 N. Fairfax Street
Suite 306
Alexandria, VA 22314
(703) 548-7790

There is a $6 fee for the information packet and directory. The center also publishes the monthly magazine *Homeopathy Today,* and offers other books and products.

The International Foundation for Homeopathy
P.O. Box 7
Edmons, WA 98020
(206) 776-4147
There is a $4 fee for the information packet and directory.

Homeopathic Educational Services
2124 Kittredge Street
Berkeley, CA 94704
(510) 649-0294

You may also want to buy homeopathic remedies for home treatment of many common ailments. The following list of manufacturers supply homeopathic remedies by mail:

The Apothecary
5415 Cedar Lane
Bethesda, MD 20814
(301) 530-0800

Apthorp Pharmacy
2201 Broadway (at 78th Street)
New York, NY 10024
(800) 775-3582
(212) 877-3480

Bailey's Pharmacy
175 Harvard Avenue
Allston, MA 02134
(800) 239-6206
(617) 782-7202

Budget Pharmacy
3001 N.W. 7th Street
Miami, FL 33125
(800) 221-9772

Boericke and Tafel, Inc.
2381 Circadian Way
Santa Rosa, CA 95407
(707) 571-8202

Dolisos America, Inc.
3014 Rigel Avenue
Las Vegas, NV 89102
(702) 871-7153

Five Elements Center
115 Route 46W
Building D. Suite 29
Mountain Lakes, NJ 07046
(201) 402-8510

Hahnemann Pharmacy
828 San Pablo Avenue
Albany, CA 94706
(510) 527-3003

Homeopathic Educational Services
2124 Kittredge Street
Berkeley, CA 94707
(510) 649-0294

Homeopathy Overnight
4111 Simon Road
Youngstown, OH 44512
(800) ARNICA-30

Humphreys Pharmacal Co.
63 Meadow Road
Rutherford, NJ 07070
(201) 933-7744

Luyties Pharmacal Co.
4200 Laclede Avenue
St. Louis, MO 63108
(800) 325-8080

Santa Monica Homeopathic Co.
629 Broadway
Santa Monica, CA 90401
(310) 395-1131

Standard Homeopathy Co.
P.O. Box 61067
154 W. 131st Street
Los Angeles, CA 90061
(213) 321-4284

Taylor's Pharmacy
230 North Park Avenue
Winter Park, FL 32789
(407) 644-1025

Washington Homeopathic Pharmacy
4914 Del Ray Avenue
Bethesda, MD 20814
(301) 656-1695

Weleda Pharmacy, Inc.
175 North Route 9W
Congers, NY 10920
(914) 268-8572

ACUPUNCTURE AND ACUPRESSURE

For more information or a referral, contact:

American Academy of Medical Acupuncture (AAMA)
5820 Wilshire Boulevard
Suite 500
Los Angeles, CA 90036
(213) 937-5514

The National Commission for the Certification of Acupuncturists (NCCA)
P.O. Box 97075
Washington, DC 20090
(202) 232-1404

For additional information on acupuncture and acupressure, as well as for a free referral to practitioners in your area, contact:

Acupressure Institute of America
1533 Shattuck Avenue
Berkeley, CA 94709
(800) 442-2232
(415) 845-1059 in California

The American Association for Acupuncture and Oriental Medicine
433 Front Street
Catasauqua, PA 18032-2506
(610) 433-2448

OTHER ORGANIZATIONS DEALING WITH ALTERNATIVE MEDICINE

Alliance for Alternatives in Health Care
P.O. Box 6279
Thousand Oaks, CA 91359-6279
(805) 494-7818

American Foundation for Alternative Health Care
25 Landfield Avenue
Monticello, NY 12701
(914) 794-8181

American Foundation of Traditional Chinese Medicine
505 Beach Street
San Francisco, CA 94133
(415) 776-0502

American Holistic Medical Association
433 Front Street
Catasauqua, PA 18032
(610) 433-2448

Committee for Freedom of Choice in Medicine
1180 Walnut Avenue
Chula Vista, CA 91911
(619) 429-8200

Complementary Medicine Networking and Referral Service
4649 Malvern
Tucson, AZ 85711
(520) 323-6291

Web Sítes of Interest

Following is a partial list of valuable medical and health sites on the
Internet:

- Dr. Marcellus Walker
  http://www.walkermd.com

- African American Health
  http://www.888Antiage.com

- Algy's Herb Page
  http://www.algy.com/herb/index.html

- The Alternative Medicine Homepage
  http://www.pitt.edu/~cbw/altm.html

- Ask Dr. Weil
  http://www.drweil.com

- Ask the Dietitian
  http://www.hoptechno.com/rdindex.htm

- Between the Lines
  http://members.aol.com/pbchowka

- "Bones Are Us"
  http://www.cosortho.com

- Detox Help
  http://www.detoxhelp.com

- Dr. Bower's Complementary and Alternative Medicine Home Page
  http://www.galen.med.virginia.edu/~pjb3s/
  ComplementaryHomePage.html

- FeMiNa: Health and Wellness
  http://www.femina.com/femina/healthandwellness

- General Complementary Medicine References
  http://www.forthrt.com/~chronicl/archiv.htm

- Harvard Health Publications
  http://www.med.harvard.edu/publications/Health_Publications

- HealthGate
  http://www.healthgate.com

- HealthWorldOnline
  http://www.healthy.net

- Homeopathic Education Services
  http://www.ihr.com/homeopat/

- Homeopathy Home Page
  http://www.dungeon.com/~cam/homeo.html

- Institute for Traditional Medicine
  http://www.europa.com/~itm

- The MedAccess Site
  http://www.medaccess.com

- MedWeb
  http://www.cc.emory.edu/WHSCL/medweb.html

- National Association of People with AIDS
  http://www.thecure.org

- NEW AGE Online
  http://www.newage.com

- OncoLink, The University of Pennsylvania Cancer
  Center Resource
  http://www.oncolink.org

- Southwest School of Botanical Medicine
  http://www.chili.rt66.com/hrbmoore/HOMEPAGE/
  HomePage.html

- Women's Medical Health Page
  http://www.bet.com/~sirlou/wmhp.html

- Yahoo!'s Alternative Medicine Page
  http://www.yahoo.com/health/alternative_medicine

- Yahoo! Health: Women's Health
  http://www.yahoo.com/health/women_s_health

What Do All Those Initials Mean?

Practitioners of natural medicine can have a number of different initials following their names. Here we spell out the meaning behind the letters:

ABMP   Associated Bodywork and Massage Professionals

AMTA   American Massage Therapy Association

AOBTA   American Oriental Bodywork Therapy Association

CA   Certified Acupuncturist

CHt   Certified Hypnotherapist

CMP   Certified Massage Practitioner

CMT   Certified Massage Therapist

DC   Doctor of Chiropractic

DHANP   Diplomate of the Homeopathic Academy of
                 Naturopathic Physicians

DipAC   Diplomate in Acupuncture

DO   Doctor of Osteopathy

DOM   Doctor of Oriental Medicine

PT	Physical Therapist
LAc, LicAc	Licensed Acupuncturist
LD	Licensed Dietitian
LMP	Licensed Massage Practitioner
LMT	Licensed Massage Therapist
MAc	Master of Acupuncture
MOM	Master of Oriental Medicine
MsT, MT	Massage Therapist
ND	Doctor of Naturopathy
NMD	Doctor of Naturopathic Medicine
OMD	Oriental Medical Doctor
RD	Registered Dietitian
RMT	Registered Massage Therapist

Index

▼

ABOUT THE AUTHORS

MARCELLUS A. WALKER, M.D., is board certified in internal medicine and licensed in acupuncture. He received his medical training at the University of Illinois School of Medicine and served his internship and residency at Duke University Medical Center. He is a member of Alpha Omega Alpha Medical Honor Society. He has served as a panel member for the National Institute of Health's position paper on acupuncture in 1997. He completed a master's degree in spiritual psychology from the University of Santa Monica and has trained in multiple disciplines of alternative medical practice. For the last decade he has been involved in the development of multidisciplinary alternative and complimentary medical centers and is currently a practitioner and corporate consultant. He is founder and medical director of the Center for Lifelong Health, a multidisciplinary group practice in New Windsor, New York, medical director of the Wayne Woodland Manor in Pennsylvania, and director of medical affairs at Nia, an African American nutrition company.

KENNETH B. SINGLETON, M.D., M.P.H., is board certified in internal medicine and holds a master's degree in public health. He received his medical training at Howard University College of Medicine and his public health training at Johns Hopkins School of Hygiene and Public Health. He served his internship at Loma Linda University Medical Center in California, and residency in internal medicine at Kettering Medical Center in Ohio. He is a member of the Alpha Omega Alpha Medical Honor Society, Med Chi of Washington, D.C., and the American Academy of Anti-Aging Medicine. He has held faculty appointments at two medical schools, Wright State University School of Medicine and Howard University College of Medicine, where he is currently a clinical assistant professor of medicine.